Mental Health Skills for Adult Nurses & Non-Specialist Healthcare Workers

Rachel Bage

Mental Health Skills for Adult Nurses & Non-Specialist Healthcare Workers

Springer

Rachel Bage
School of Health and Care Sciences
University of Lincoln
Lincoln, UK

ISBN 978-3-032-32834-2 ISBN 978-3-032-32835-9 (eBook)
https://doi.org/10.1007/978-3-032-32835-9

This Springer imprint is published by the registered company Springer Nature Switzerland AG
The registered company address is: Gewerbestrasse 11, 6330 Cham, Switzerland

To Arthur—the little boy who made me a Mummy.

To Eliza—my twin, and strong-willed little girl. I couldn't love you both anymore.

To Alan—for supporting me in every crazy thing I do.

Preface

Those working in adult and child settings encounter mental distress every day—whether supporting service users with long-term conditions, caring for those in acute crisis or working alongside families coping with illness, loss and uncertainty. This book begins with a simple truth: mental health is everyone's business. It is not just for those in mental health specialist services.

We are working and living in a complicated world. Cost of living crises, increasing demands on family life, wars and conflict, and technological and AI advances amongst other challenges makes the world a confusing and challenging place. We are seeing increasing levels of poor mental health across the world.

Adult nurses and practitioners are often the first professionals to recognise signs of distress. Those working in the adult field are often the first professionals in contact. Mental health conditions, such as depression, substance misuse and anxiety often, coexist with physical illness and impact how people can access care, adhere to treatment programmes and experience recovery. However, many non-specialist practitioners feel unprepared, uncertain or underconfident when addressing service users' mental health needs. This is often more apparent in fast-paced and high-pressure environments such as Accident and Emergency. The lack of alignment between responsibility and preparedness reflects wider challenges within modern healthcare systems. However, it also offers an opportunity for meaningful change in the way we view physical and mental health together.

I have seen significant change within my own tine in the profession. It was once commonplace to see service users referred to as "one of yours". It is still joked that mental health nurses are not proper nurses. However, we have now started to work together much closer, although there remains much work to do. We have seen changes in the way our students approach the topic too—with a focus on holistic care. My own employer, a post 92-university, has recently developed a compulsory module on mental health for adult nursing students, and another shared module with mental health and child nursing students. These are small steps in the right direction, and I couldn't be prouder to be involved in it.

This book is written to support adult nurses, physiotherapist, occupational therapists, speech and language practitioners and other practitioners to bridge the gap. These clinicians do not need to become experts, but this book hopes to strengthen confidence, knowledge and compassion in responding to mental health needs seen daily. We all need to take small steps to growing our confidence and knowledge. I know when I worked in practice, I wish I knew more about adult health, and I am sure that feeling is shared the other way round.

This book draws on contemporary evidence, models and structures, and nursing values. There are case studies and reflective prompts throughout to offer opportunity for critical thinking and to aid the connect between theory and practice. Every chapter offers a summary of key learning points for your practice. This book hopes to make you curious about mental health practice, and fundamentally, eager to know more.

Lincoln, UK Rachel Bage

Contents

The Background of Physical Health and Mental Health

Case Study 1

Jack is a patient who has been admitted to A + E with sepsis, secondary to pneumonia. His observations have started to improve, but he remains restless and he has not settled at all in the 12 hours he has been in A + E. He has been stopped from pulling at his wires and drips several times throughout the morning.

As the nurse approached, he is shouting 'let me out' and 'they are watching me'. He looks tired and unsettled. Jack tells the nurse that he is not safe here and he needs to go home.

What do you think is the nurse's role in supporting Jack?
How would you approach supporting Jack whilst he is in the A + E Department?

Why Mental Health Is Everyone's Business

Mental health is a fundamental part of our overall wellbeing, influencing how we behave, think and feel. Mental health impacts all of us—families, schools, universities, communities, workplaces and entire nations. The way we view mental health, mental ill health, and mental health services has changed monumentally in the last 100 years. Even in recent history, change has been vast.

Mental health, or mental ill health, continues to cause issue to the UK, and the world. All of us will know people who are impacted with mental ill health, and 1/5 will will have suffered a common mental health condition ourselves in the last year (Liubertiene et al. 2025). The most common mental health conditions within the UK are generalised anxiety disorder, panic attacks and depression (Liubertiene et al. 2025). Suicide rates in the UK are increasing in both males and females.

The situation is similar globally. The World Health Organisation estimates that at least one billion people globally are living with a mental health condition (WHO

R. Bage, *Mental Health Skills for Adult Nurses & Non-Specialist Healthcare Workers*, https://doi.org/10.1007/978-3-032-32835-9_1

2025). Mental ill health affects people of all social classes, ages and income levels (WHO 2025). In 2021, nearly 750,000 people internationally ended their life by suicide (WHO 2022). A recent global study found that approximately half of the population will have experienced one or more diagnosable mental health condition by the age of 75 (McGrath et al. 2023).

The cost of this high level of ill mental health shows in NHS usage. In 2023, approximately 3.8 million people were in contact with mental health, learning disability or autism services (NHS England 2024). Within this, 1 in five girls aged 16 are in contact with these services, and more than one million children (NHS England 2024). In the 21/22 year, approximately 8% of NHS funding went towards mental health services. Whilst funding has been increasing, there are still not enough services to cope with this demand (Gilburt and Mallorie 2024a, b). Mental health services are provided from some of the oldest estates within the UK, with around 18% constructed before the NHS existed, and classified as not suitable for use (Gilburt and Mallorie 2024b).

Mental health directly affects physical health. Poor mental health can impact physical health such as heart disease, immune systems and diabetes. Chronic ill health can cause the development of depression or anxiety. When mental health is neglected, healthcare systems face greater strain, and recovery from physical illness becomes more difficult. By caring about mental health at a societal level, communities can improve overall health outcomes and reduce long-term healthcare costs.

We also know the relationship between work and mental health which is bidirectional. Good mental health is key in finding a job and retaining a job (Wilson and Finch 2021). Equally, mental health is impacted by unemployment and can be a contributing cause to conditions such as depression, anxiety and lower self-esteem (Wilson and Finch 2021). Having a job is good for our mental health. ONS figures suggest that every year 300,000 people leave employment due to poor mental health (ONS 2025). Recent research has suggested that poor mental health costs UK employers at least £51 billion per year (Deloitte 2024). Poor mental health costs all of us by reducing the working population year on year.

Stigma is another reason mental health must be everyone's concern. Increasing interest by key figures is also heightening the focus internationally of mental health. Prince William, Kate Middleton, Simone Biles and Harry Wales are all people who have either spoken publicly or worked to highlight mental health challenges. Celebrity and well-known suicides such as Graham Thorpe, Caroline Flack and Thomas Kingston have highlighted the perils of mental ill health. Reducing stigma requires collective effort—through education, open conversations and positive representation in media. It is now rarely the case that a story about mental health is not in the contemporary media.

Historically, mental health and physical health have been viewed very differently within the United Kingdom (UK). However, there is increasing focus on providing care for the whole person following the introduction of UK's Health and Social Care Act (2012). Parity of esteem, or the principle that mental health must be given an equal priority to physical health, is a principle enshrined in UK law. Parity looks at ideas such as increasing access to services, parity of treatments and 24/7 services.

We know there is also increasing clinical crossover. Research shows that between 23 and 42% of older people admitted to an acute hospital have a diagnosis of dementia (de Vries et al. 2019). Mental health service users are often left with little choice but to attend emergency departments out of hours due to the lack of mental health services (CQC 2018). Every clinician will work with somebody who has a mental health diagnosis, and it is not just a role for mental health nurses.

Jack's Case

With Jack, the nurse's role would be to reorientate and comfort Jack. As we work in these environments, it can be easy to forget how scary and unsettling these environments can be. It would be even more unsettling to have a drip, drip stand and the noise associated with these.

In approaching Jack, staff need to ensure they are approaching Jack so that he can see you, and you are not startling him in any way. It is always good practice to ensure you start to orientate him by introducing yourself and your role. You should also make sure on every interaction that you remind him where he is.

At this point, it may also be useful to get some sort of baseline for Jack. Jack may have a relative there with him, or you may need to ring a relative or care provider (if he consents to this). This is all useful information to gather even whilst he is unwell, so you can understand where his baseline is, and what you are aiming for.

In Jack's case, it is very clear that the A + E environment is not going to be beneficial for his physical and mental health. Jack would be a good candidate for a frailty ward, where the ward design and environment will have been better designed for someone like Jack. In my own local department, that involved coloured bays and extra-coloured doors to help reorientate people.

A Short History of Mental Health Care

Hospitals Before Psychiatry

Prior to the development of psychiatry, and the institutions this brought, societies treated mental ill health within family structures, the wider community or religious settings. Little specialised care existed. Mental ill health, and wider ill health, was often viewed in the lens of spirituality or moral interpretations, and the severely ill were often banished from the community to live in solitude with family.

Bimaristans

Jundi—Shapur, meaning 'beautiful garden', was a city in Khuzistan, in south-western Persia. A university, medical school and hospital were established in about 555 AD within Jundi—Shapur. This was the first hospital type establishment. It took the philosophical and medical traditions from a range of cultures including Persians, Greeks, Indians, Zoroastrians, Jews and Nestorians. During the Abbasid Caliphate, the capital was moved to Baghdad in 762 AD, where the successful treatment of Caliph Abu Jaifar Al-Mansur by Jirjis ibn Bukhtyishu led to the establishment of the first bimaristan (hospital) by his son under Caliph Harun Al-Rashid. Baghdad subsequently became a major centre of political, scientific, and medical innovation, with numerous hospitals contributing to the Golden Age of Islamic medicine (Miller 2006).

Bimaristans came in two types—fixed and mobile (Miller 2006). Mobile bimaristans were the older of the two and were believed to date back to the time of the Prophet Muhammed. During the Ghazwah Kandaq, or Battle of the Ditch, a separate tent was established for the wounded. These only developed further and were often staffed with doctors and pharmacists. These 'field hospitals' were well equipped with instruments, tents, and doctors, nurses and orderlies. They allowed services to reach more rural communities and those who were disabled and disadvantaged (Miller 2006).

It is not so clear about the development of fixed bimaristans. There is still disagreement about the first, either Ummayad Caliph Al-Walid bin Abdel Malik in 707 AD, or Caliph Harun Al-Rashid later in 786–809 AD. These bimaristans were chosen to be in the best locations, atop of hilltops or along rivers. Al-Adudi Hospital in Baghdad was known to be close to the river, allowing the river to flow through its courtyard and halls (Miller 2006). Al-Mansuri Hospital was constructed in Cairo in 1284 AD and became the prototype for many of the further hospitals. With a capacity of 8000, it served citizens regardless of colour, religion, sex, age or social status. Service users stayed until they were fully recovered or transferred to the convalescent ward to regain their strength (Miller 2006). Wards were equal but separated by gender and there were wards to medicine, surgery, fever, wounds and eye diseases. These were the first sites known to have separate wards for mania. Hospitals were well equipped with pharmacies, libraries, lecture halls, mosques and occasionally chapels. Service users had access to musicians and musical therapy (Miller 2006).

Bimaristans were also thought to be the birth of the written record. Students were used to write notes and keep records of treatments and service users. However, mental health care is frequently viewed through the lens of the asylum system, despite the fact that its origins extend beyond these institutions.

Asylums

Reflective Questions

What are your thoughts and feelings about how care was provided in asylums?

What might daily life have felt like for people living in asylums, and how does that challenge the way we think about 'care' today?

What does this reveal about society's treatment of people who fall outside dominant social norms?

In 1247, the Priory of St Mary of Bethlehem was founded, focussed to healing sick paupers. It first was established as a very small site and later became known as the Bethlehem Hospital. The Bethlehem Hospital, sometimes shortened to Bedlam, was on the site of London Liverpool Street Hospital. At some point in its history, monks began to accept service users who had symptoms of mental ill health rather than physical disease. By 1403, 'lunatic' service users were the majority of Bethlem's service user group—and the first mental institution was founded (Historic England 2019). It was taken over by the City of London in 1346 and by this point was known to take service users with mental ill health, learning disabilities, epilepsy and dementia. At this point in Bedlem, the daily routine was largely punishment and religious devotion. We know from the hospital inventory that service users had chains, manacles and locks and stocks (Historic England 2019).

By the 1750s, the UK had only three public asylums in England and one each in Scotland and Ireland. These housed no more than 400 inmates each and served a population of people called 'lunatics'. Private madhouses were also established at this point, but these served only a small population. At this point, most mentally unwell service users remained in their family homes or another domestic setting (Houston 2019). The first large asylum was built in the early 1800s within the UK. One of the earliest asylums was the Middlesex County Lunatic Asylum, on the outskirts of London, and set the standard for future developments (Science Museum 2018).

Lincoln Lunatic Asylum was an asylum opened in 1820. It was a purpose-built asylum in central Lincoln. Lincoln is known for being the first asylum to be run without use of mechanical restraints, under the leadership of Edward Parker Charlesworth and Robert Hill (Eleanor Glanville Institute n.d.). This was thought to happen in the year 1837, and this work was then seen across other institutes such as the Hanwell Asylum in Middlesex (BBC 2025).

The 1930s saw the first change in the asylums. The 1930 Mental Health Treatment Act saw the word 'asylum' replaced by 'mental hospital'. However, there was little move away from the big old mental institutions until the 1950s (Sidi 2021). Institutionalisation hit a peak in the 1950s, with approximately 150,000 people in the UK within an asylum (Houston 2019). At this point, there was increasing will to close long stay psychiatric wards. Enoch Powell, health minister, made his famous 'water towers' speech in 1961, promising a reduction in hospital beds over a 15-year period. Instead, discharge was far faster than this (Sidi 2021). Deinstitutionalisation was made statutory law in 1990, with the introduction of the NHS and Community Offenders. This saw the final stages of the asylum closure, with responsibility of the care of long term mentally ill service users moved to Local Authority Care. This Act had huge impacts on the boundaries between health and social care and offered massive restructuring to the care system (Sidi 2021). The final large-scale asylum closures happened by the year 2000. Lincoln Asylum, for example, closed in 1988 (Eleanor Glanville Institute n.d.).

Viewpoints of Mental Health

Sociological Understandings of Mental Health

Sociological approaches regard mental health and illness as an aspect of their social circumstances. Sociological approaches may look at social conditions such as stress, negative life events or social support. Equally, sociologists may focus on social and cultural influences affect the response and definitions of mental ill health in our communities (Horwitz 2012).

Since the nineteenth century, mental disorder was traced to observations across asylums. At this point, many of the ideas were linked to traumatic impacts of warfare (Pilgrim and McKeown 2024). The work of Emile Durkheim, Suicide, was thought of as the first sociological study into mental health (Horwitz 2012).

The assumption of social causationists is that psychiatric disorders are real and the work of empirical sociologists is to trace the social forces that make contributions to aetiology (Pilgrim and McKeown 2024). Sociologists focus on the impact of social circumstances on mental health, such as life events or social structures. They assume that different individuals in the same circumstances will have a similar level of mental health or ill health (Horwitz 2012).

Critical Psychological Ideas

Psychological understandings of mental health and distress are used to develop interventions and understanding of mental ill health (Bentall and McKeown 2024). Psychology looks at the relationships between thoughts, feelings and behaviours. This background of understanding has helped to develop therapies such as cognitive behavioural therapy, person-centred counselling and psychodynamic therapy (Bentall and McKeown 2024).

Mental health nurses will normally receive some background in psychology during their degrees but will likely not have studied psychology on its own. If mental health practitioners wish to go on to deliver therapies, they will study this as an added course or training module (Bentall and McKeown 2024). There is an argument that mental health nurses should study more psychology and psychological therapies as part of their degree, especially as A-Level or College-level psychology is often one of the persuaders for young people signing up for the mental health nursing degree. Talking therapies practitioners' study separately.

Philosophical Understanding of Mental Health

The philosophy of mental health looks at issues concerning mental illness, health and healthcare. It encourages investigation of the world prior to the establishment of empirical methods and thus before the invention of science (Thornton 2024).

Philosophy played a large role in assisting our elders and ancestors who were literate in managing those who were unwell with poor mental health, and we can still see some of those early teachings within manuscripts and teaching. Some key contributors for the philosophical approach for mental health include Goethe, Voltaire, Hippocrates, Aristotle, Cicero and Nietzsche (Allin 2024).

Psychiatric Understanding of Mental Health

Psychiatric practice has been deemed controversial by some. Thibaut (2018) highlights the discussions around diagnostic criteria of psychiatric diseases and the subjectivity of clinical assessment. Kinderman (2014) argues that mental health should be delivered as a non-medical practice, and the biological aspects of mental health care should be seen as the minority care within mental health. Kinderman argued that most presentations are psychosocial.

Psychiatrists have also become concerned over recent years that their position may be taken over by other professionals (Double 2024). Equally, there is debate about the value of mental health medication (Double 2024). However, in recent times it is clear that psychiatrists have stayed very much involved in the provision of mental health care.

Reflective Questions
What do you think is your viewpoint of mental health?
Are there any of the views you particularly agree or disagree with?

The Structural Divide: Funding, Policy and Systems

Reflective Questions
Where do you think people fall through due to structural divides?
How do hospital policies or care pathways support integrated care—or reinforce separation?

The history of recent mental health in the UK follows two main paths: the rise of psychopharmacology and a focus of deinstitutionalisation (Turner et al. 2015). The 1959 Mental Health Act and the 1962 Hospital Plan led to the closure of the asylums and the move of psychiatric care into the wider hospital systems (Turner et al. 2015). This alongside the development of antipsychotic drugs and mood stabilisers during the latter 1950s allowed an increased number of service users to be treated in the community (Mental Health Foundation 2019).

1959—Mental Health Act

The Mental Health Act was implemented following the report *of the Royal Commission on the law relating to mental deficiency* (the Percy report—1959). This Act repeals the 1890 Act and abolishes the Board of Control. This was a significant change from earlier legislation and moved more towards the provision of treatment rather than just institutionalisation (Mental Health Foundation 2019).

1961—Enoch Powell's Speech

The renowned 1961 speech labelled the 'Water tower speech' signals the closure of the large mental asylums across the UK. In this period there were significant staff shortages, particularly in the nursing field (Hulatt 2014). Hospitals were being forced to accept unsuitable recruits which impacted quality of care (Hulatt 2014).

1962—Hospital Plan

Enoch Powell's speech led to the development of the *A Hospital Plan for England and Wales.* This plan looked to establish small-scale psychiatric inpatient units in District General Hospitals, with the local authorities offering the range of community services (Mental Health Foundation 2019).

1971—Psychiatry

1971 saw the establishment of the Royal College of Psychiatrists, established from the Royal Medico-Psychological Association (Mental Health Foundation 2019).

1974—NHS Reorganisation

NHS reorganisation means that mental health services are combined with general medical and hospital services into local NHS districts with the local authorities (Mental Health Foundation 2019).

1975—Butler Report

The Butler Report, titled *Report of the Committee on Mentally Abnormal Offenders* Cmnd 6244, was published (Mental Health Foundation 2019).

1983—Mental Health Act

The new Mental Health Act (1983) was published. This strengthened the civil rights for mentally unwell service users (Mental Health Foundation 2019).

1988—Griffiths Report

The Griffiths report, titled *Community care: agenda for action* was published. This led to changes in policy and the 1990 NHS and Community Care Act (Mental Health Foundation 2019).

1990—Community Care Act

The Community Care Act led to the introduction of the care programme approach (CPA). This provides an effective framework for mental health care for people with severe mental health problem (Mental Health Foundation 2019).

1991-96—NHS Trusts

Between 1991 and 96, NHS Trusts were established. Within this, separate Mental Health Trusts were established (Mental Health Foundation 2019).

1992—Reed Report

The Reed Report, titled *Review of health and social services for mentally disordered offenders and others requiring similar services*, was published.

1998—Modernising Mental Health

The *Modernising Mental Health* white paper was released. This was the first comprehensive government statement re the direction of policy within mental health services since 1975 (Mental Health Foundation 2019).

1999—National Service Framework

1999 saw the establishment of the National Service Framework (NSF) for adult mental health services. This was a 10-year plan for the development of mental health services for adults of working age, with similar developments within Scotland and Wales (Mental Health Foundation 2019). The key services introduced within the MSF were assertive outreach teams, crisis resolution and home treatment teams and early intervention teams (Mental Health Foundation 2019).

2001—Development of an Institute

The development of the National Institute for Mental Health in England was established to support service development (Mental Health Foundation 2019).

2003—Death of Rocky Bennett

The Blofeld Inquiry was published following the death of David 'Rocky' Bennett which highlighted to problems with service provision for black and minority ethnic groups.

2006—Older People Mental Health

In 2006 the paper *everybody's business: integrated mental health services for older adults* which was the first integrated policy statement for mental health within older adults.

2007—Mental Health Act

The new Mental Health Act was published after discussions between the government and the *Mental Health Alliance*. The most controversial development in this was the establishment on Community Treatment Orders (CTOs). CTOs allow service users who have been discharged from hospital to be required to accept treatment when outside the hospital or face the risk of being recalled to hospital (Mental Health Foundation 2019).

2009—New Government Strategy

The Government strategy was outlined in *New horizons: towards a shared vision for mental health* which prioritised equality, personalisation, equality and stigma, and the physical health of service users with a mental health condition (Department of Health 2009).

2011—No Health Without Mental Health

The Cross-government publication *No health without mental health* introduced a changed focus on public health, and improving outcomes (Parliament 2026).

2016—Five Year Forward View for Mental Health

This is an an independent strategy setting out how the NHS in England should transform mental health services (NHS England 2016).

2019—Long-Term Plan

The NHS Long Term Plan was published in 2019. It aimed to develop new integrated mental health community teams for adults with severe mental health illnesses (NHS 2019).

2024—Darzi Report

Lord Darzi's report, *Independent investigation of the National Health Service in England.*

2025—Mental Health Bill

The Mental Health Bill received Royal Assent in later 2025. The Bill delivers on the desire to give service users greater choice and autonomy, with enhanced rights.

A shift of focus has been seen throughout the last 100 years in mental health practice. Services have moved from rights and recovery to a focus on risk and safety, modernisation and overall wellbeing (Mental Health Foundation 2019).

Current Picture

Activity

What does your local provider look like for mental health services?

Over the last 10 years, there has been a significant shift in the architecture of NHS Providers. There has been a push towards larger trusts and trusts sharing board-level leadership (NHS Confederation 2024). Many of these mergers have involved community and mental health trusts, and larger mental health trusts have also been established (NHS Confederation 2024). This has happened not on a national drive, but more for local reasons and the drive of individual leaders (NHS Confederation 2024).

There are currently 252 NHS providers. Of this, there are currently 19 mental health providers and 29 combined mental health and learning disability and community providers (NHS Providers 2025b).

Commissioning

One of the biggest structural divides exists due to funding inequalities in mental health services. Currently, most mental health services are commissioned by local Integrated Care Boards. Commissioning comprises activities such as: assessing needs priority setting, planning, procuring of services and monitoring quality (Kings Fund 2024). However, some very specialist mental health services are commissioned by NHS England, e.g. children's services. NHS England is currently working to give delegating responsibility for commissioning mental health, learning disability and autism services to NHS-Led Provider Collaboratives. NHS-Led Provider Collaboratives are groups of specialist providers, with a lead provider, that will work together to manage budget and care pathways within populations (Garratt 2024; Wickens 2022). Most local mental health services are not ring-fenced, and the Integrated Care Boards are able to determine mental health budget from its overall allocation. NHS England not the government does not have the control to specify how much funding goes to mental health services locally (Garratt 2024; Wickens 2022). However, local areas must meet the 'mental health investment standard' (MHIS), which means local mental health spending has to be as large proportionally as overall increase is in the local health funding (Garratt 2024). NHS England reports that this requirement has been met since 2015/16 (Garratt 2024). The total planned spend on MHIS in 2025/26 was £13.671 billion.

The way services are funded further highlights systematic differences between mental and physical health. Adult physical health sectors offer activity-based payments. Activity-based payments mean that providers are paid based on the amount and type of care delivered. This allows services to offer some alignment between funding and demand. Mental health services are largely funded through block contracts, which allocate a fixed budget regardless of fluctuations in demands. Block contracts have been criticised for many reasons: lack of transparency about spending, the masking of underfunding and whether services meet local demand. Capital investment for mental health infrastructure, such as buildings, has also lagged in mental health services.

Activity

Look through your own local mental health, adult and learning disability services. How are these commissioned? Do you have more than one trust for these services, or are they provided by the same trust?

Workforce

Recruitment and retention remain persistent challenges in both adult and mental health services. Mental health services continue to have significant staffing challenges especially across psychiatrists, nurses and psychological therapists. However, the workforce has increased since 2010, with nurse levels increasing by 3% and therapists and support services increasing by nearer 50% (Gilburt and Mallorie 2024a).

However, evidence has shown that there has been uneven expansion across the sector. The greatest increase in psychiatry staffing has been in general psychiatry, whereas older adult psychiatry and learning disability services have repeatedly been unable to fill vacant positions (Kings Fund 2024). Other areas in mental health have also struggled, with persistent child and adolescent (CAMHS) psychiatrist vacancies despite an increase in overall number, and AMHP numbers not increasing in the last 5 years (Gilbert and Mallorie 2024a).

Vacancies remain high in mental health services. In 2023, across every region, vacancy levels in mental health services were higher than other NHS services. Challenges can be particularly acute in some areas, such as inpatient mental health services (Gilbert and Mallorie 2024a).

Activity

What aspects of historical provision exist in your area? Think about policies, attitudes and pathways?

Physical–Mental Health Interdependence

Modern medicine is increasingly seeing the relationship between mind and body.

Background

The mortality gap in mental health refers to the life expectancy difference between people living with severe mental illness (SMI) and the general population. The current research persistently highlights that this gap is between 15 and 20 years—this cuts life shorter than diabetes, obesity and smoking (King's College 2025).

Data from the NHS suggests that of recent years, 66% of people with a severe mental illness who died prematurely died of a preventable physical health condition such as respiratory disease, heart disease and liver disease (NHS England 2014).

People with a serious mental illness are:

6.6 times increased risk of respiratory disease.
6.5 times increased risk of liver disease.
4.1 times increased risk of cardiovascular disease.
People with a serious mental illness are twice as likely to smoke (NHS England 2025).

Historical Context

Western medicine has long considered that the mind and body are separate entities (Jayasinghe 2002). Indeed, it can be traced back to work of Descartes, a renaissance philosopher, in the sixteenth century, who discussed the concept of mind-body dualism (Bennett 2024; Ventriglio and Bhugra 2015). Other cultures have often seen the mind-body as much closer (e.g. Ayurveda and Vedic systems). The biomedical model of illness became the norm, something we now think of as reductionist in nature (Bennett 2024).

Work has been ongoing to realign this thinking of the mind and body and to see the body as a complex physiological system combining mind and body (Bennett 2024). Evidence now shows that the mind and body are inextricably linked. There remain relatively few models that fully integrate physical and mental illness. Researchers now call for better integration of services between mental and physical health and parity in funding for research in both fields (Ventriglio and Bhugra 2015).

How Physical Health Impacts Each Other

Work by Ohrnberger et al. (2017) has adapted an economic framework to look at two components of the health capital—physical and mental health. This helps to theorise several channels in which physical and mental health may impact on each other. This framework is shown in Fig. 1.

Chronic Illness and Emotional Burden

Chronic illness covers some of the most prevalent conditions in the UK, such as diabetes, heart disease and chronic obstructive pulmonary disease. These are often managed long term, rather than curable. It is currently estimated that more than four million people in England who have a long-term physical health condition also have a mental health condition. Forty percent of people with depression and anxiety have a concurrent long-term condition (NHS England 2025). Many of these subsequently experience poorer health outcomes and reduced quality of life (Naylor et al. 2012).

Chronic illness also impacts a person as a whole. In 2023, eight million people aged between 16 and 64 reported having a long-term health condition that limits the type of amount of work they could do (The Health Foundation 2024).

Biological Pathways

Stress Response System

Stress contributes to a higher chance of developing mental health problems (Kantor and Vuletić 2023). Repeated stress has also been linked to high blood pressure, obesity and brain changes contributing to anxiety, depression and anxiety (Harvard

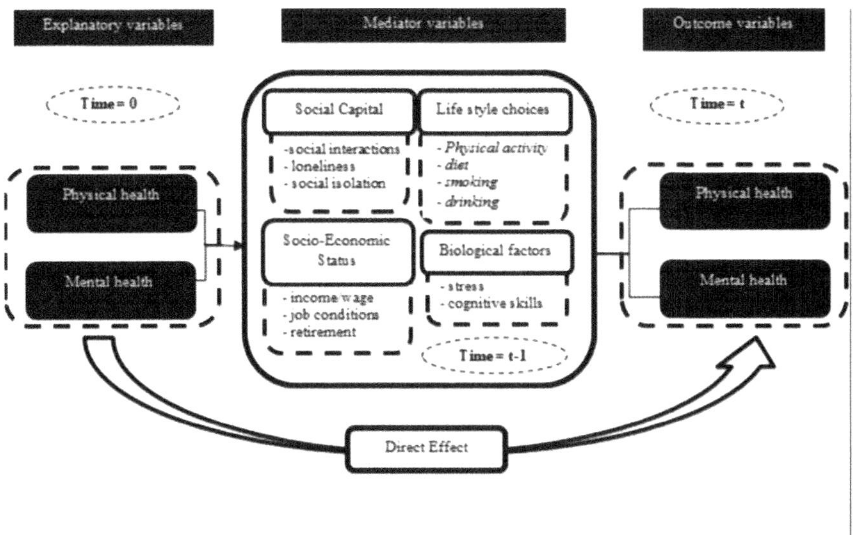

Fig. 1 Direct and indirect effects between physical and mental health. (From Science Direct, Elsevier, https://www.sciencedirect.com/science/article/pii/S0277953617306639, licenced under CC-BY 4.0)

Health 2011). Stress has long been a focus in neuroscience (Ghasemi et al. 2024). Any disruption to the body's equilibrium causes a stress response, with the associated psychological and behavioural modifications (Ghasemi et al. 2024). Activation of the stress responses involves activation of sympathetic nervous system and the hypothalamic-pituitary-adrenal (HPA) axis and the fight/flight/freeze responses (Mifsud and Reul 2018).

The stress response system has three main biological functions: to coordinate the allostatic response to physical and psychosocial challenges; to encode and filter information about the organism's social and physical environment; and to regulate the organism's physiology and behaviour in areas such as defensive behaviours, competitive risk-taking, learning and reproductive functioning (Del Giudice et al. 2011). All of us will have different tolerances to stress. Some people are able to cope with a great amount of stress in our lives. Others can tolerate very little. In Fig. 2, you can see the theory of the Adaptive Calibration Model (ACM), a development of the stress response theory. This model offers a framework to understand the individual differences in responsivity and developmental trajectories leading to the differences. In this theory, authors suggest that individual difference in stress responsivity is largely due to the result of conditional adaptation—which is the evolved ability of an organism to modify the developmental trajectory to match local conditions of the environment (Del Giudice et al. 2011).

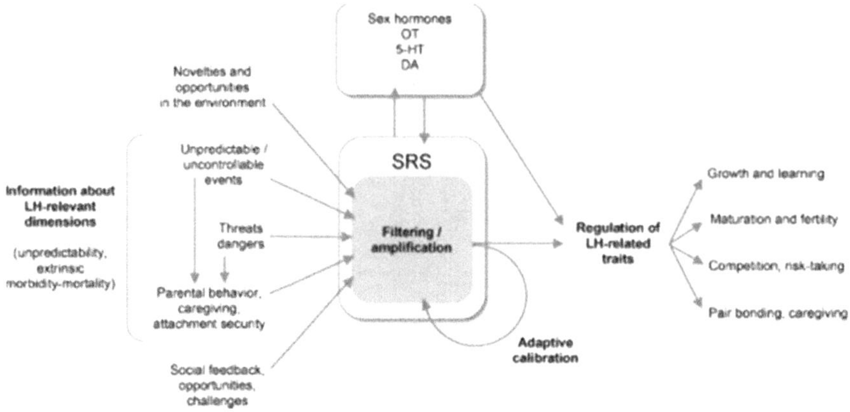

Fig. 2 Conceptual structure of the Adaptive Calibration Model (Del Giudice et al. 2011)

Inflammation Theory

Evidence is building that inflammation is a risk factor for mental illnesses (Clesse et al. 2022). Figure 3 gives a good explanation of the current thoughts around inflammation's role in mental ill health (Yin et al. 2024). In this hypothesis, psychoneuroimmunological dysfunctions are thought to be key, with a number of areas of inflammation being linked, which can be seen in Fig. 3. This is based on findings in those with severe depression—subsets have altered peripheral immune systems, cytokines may impact neurotransmitter metabolism, neuroendocrine function and brain activity, acute administration of cytokines causes sickness behaviour (with similar features to depression) and people having cytokine treatment develop depression symptoms (Zunszain et al. 2012).

There are a number of key strategies for treatment that are currently being linked to anti-inflammatories and depression:

1. Non-steroidal anti-inflammatory drugs.
2. Selective COX-2 Inhibition.
3. Non-selective COX inhibition.
4. Cytokine modulators.
5. Omega-3 polysaturated fatty acids.
6. Minocycline.
7. Statins.
8. Probiotics and prebiotics.
9. Physical exercise (Yin et al. 2024).

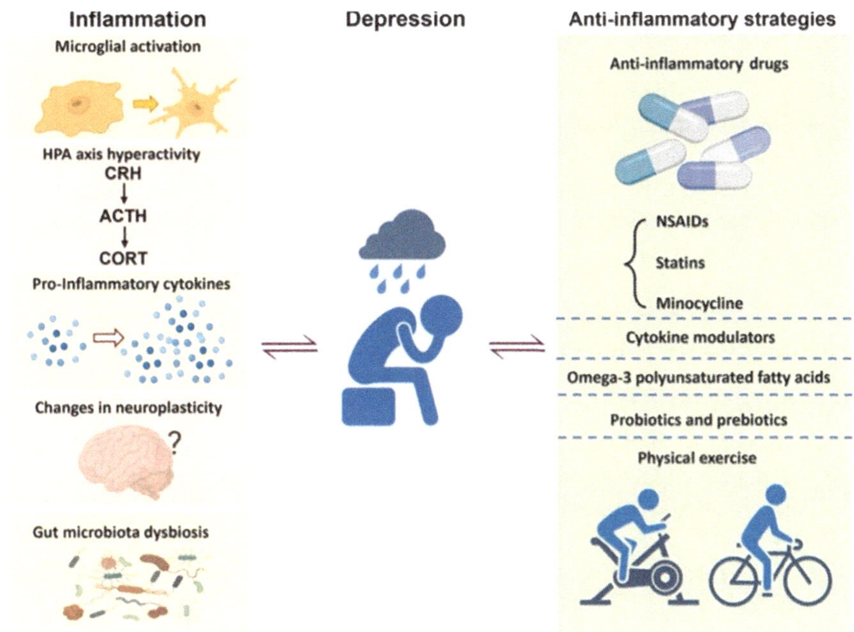

Fig. 3 Depression and inflammation

How Mental Health Impacts Physical Health?

Behavioural Pathways

Mental health is often linked to lifestyle choices such as physical activity, smoking, diet and alcohol consumption (Ohrnberger et al. 2017; Bourke et al. 2025). Participating in healthy lifestyle behaviours may play an important role in the management and treatment of mental health conditions (Bourke et al. 2025). A study looking at data from the UK Biobank examined 290,000 people's data, which found that there were seven healthy lifestyle factors linked with a lower risk of depression which were:

- Moderate alcohol consumption.
- Healthy diet.
- Regular physical activity.
- Healthy sleep.
- Never smoking.
- Low-to-moderate sedentary behaviour.
- Frequent social connection (Zhao et al. 2023).

Ohrnberger et al. (2017) found that physical activity is the most important factor in the relationship between physical health and mental health.

Stress

It likely comes as no surprise that stress is thought to play a role in the development of mental ill health. Stress influences a person's health behaviours. A systematic review completed found that stress is more likely linked to unhealthier behaviours (Bamert et al. 2025). Pathophysiological consequences of chronic stress include immune system deregulation, cardiovascular disease and other health problems (Ghasemi et al. 2024).

Social and Environmental Factors

Case Study 2

A 65-year-old woman, Alix, has attended A + E 18 times in the last 6 months. She has a diagnosis of COPD and depression. A + E staff have become frustrated with her constant attendances, with little progress being made.

What is the role of mental health services, and what is the role of physical health services?

How should they be working together?

Annual Physical Health Checks

Anyone with a diagnosis of schizophrenia, bipolar disorder or psychosis should be offered a yearly physical health check with their general practitioner (GP), or the physical health team within their local mental health trust. This check should look at the following components at a minimum:

- Alcohol consumption status.
- Blood glucose or HbA1c test (as clinically appropriate).
- Blood pressure.
- Body mass index.
- Lipid profile.
- Smoking status (NHS England 2025).

Some services are commissioned to provide a more extensive physical health check for service users. This comprises all, or some, of the following:

- Medical and family history.
- Blood-borne virus and liver function screening.
- Cardiovascular risk assessment (including QRisk).
- Relevant national immunisation programmes.
- Support to access relevant national screening programmes, including cancer screening.

- Oral health advice and brief interventions.
- Assessment of physical activity levels.
- Sexual and reproductive health assessment and advice (including contraception).
- Substance use assessment.
- Medicines reconciliation and monitoring.

The proportion of people currently receiving this annual health check varies between 60% and 82% (NHS England 2025).

Reflective Questions

Who is best placed to deliver physical health checks for service users with serious mental illness. Should this be the role of mental health services, or primary care services?

Why?

Case Study

With Alix, working together is crucial for Alix and professionals to feel more supported. If Alix is yet to be referred to hospital-based mental health services, arranging this may be a useful first step. For most trusts, Mental Health Liaison Services is the first step for accessing mental health services.

We know there is significant crossover in many physical health conditions, and COPD is one of those conditions where the crossover is well documented. COPD services may offer their own mental health professionals, or access to cognitive behavioural therapy. A multidisciplinary team meeting should be arranged, to try and establish a list of priorities for Alix if a role for mental health services has been identified.

Stigma, Language and Professional Identity

Nine out of 10 people with mental health problems say that they are impacted negatively by stigma and discrimination. People with a mental health condition are one of the least likely groups to find work, be in a steady relationship, live in suitable accommodation and be socially included within their communities (Mental Health Foundation 2021).

The History of Stigma

Stigmatisation of the mental ill health has long been the case, and the word 'stigmatisation' comes along with negative connotations. For example, Ancient Greece saw the word 'stigma' used to brand criminals. For many generations, and arguably even through to today, society has not treated some people with mental illness better than criminals. In fact, in many parts of the world today, they continue to be imprisoned (Rössler 2016). Mental illness has also long been intertwined with religion—thought to be a punishment of God, and something we will discuss further in chapter 'Inclusivity' (Rössler 2016).

Here in the UK, the first programme screened about mental illness was in 1857, called The Hurt Mind, and featured people from a Hospital in Croydon. They spoke about their experiences of mental distress. Much controversy was caused following the airing of this, due to the power of psychiatrists in the programme, and the biased discussion regarding physical treatments of mental illness. It was maybe the first opportunity for many, who had not experienced mental health in their own lives, to see experiences of people living with mental illness (Selby 2020).

Anti-stigma campaigns and the growing social media campaigns have perhaps gone some way to changing views about mental illness. Most recently, Prince William opened up about his own mental health and the role of male role models on BBC Radio One (BBC 2026). Prior to this, Harry Windsor and Meghan Markle have spoken very publicly about mental health on social media and within mainstream media.

Equally, previous Governments have made numerous commitments to reduce stigma and discrimination in regards to mental ill health. Strategies have included 'No Health Without Mental Health', which included reducing stigma as one of its six key objectives. The 2014 campaign 'Closing the gap: Essential priorities for mental health' also highlighted the end of discrimination as one of its key objectives. Much remains in the literature around 'parity of esteem' and ensuring the same care for physical and mental health.

Inclusive Language in Mental Health

Reflective Questions

What negative language have you heard within your own workplaces?
Do you challenge this language use? What stops you from challenging it?

The way we use language matters. Generations of people have grown up in communities which have used words like 'psycho', 'schizo', 'nuts', 'loony' and 'crazy' (Mental Health Foundation 2019). Working in practice, I heard things from other professionals like 'one of yours' on a regular occasion. The way we use our words affects how people seek help, and it can make people think they are 'suffering' from something or make them feel less of their community (Mental Health Foundation 2019).

There will always be debate on precisely the right words to use. This is much like the debate on how to refer to our service users—we may use patient, service user or client. However, there is agreement that we should be moving to a more person-centred approach (McCormack and McCance 2006). This means we are moving from a schizophrenic person to a person with schizophrenia. These are small changes, but they show that the illness is only one aspect of that person's life (Volkow et al. 2021).

We should also consider how we use terminology that implied a negative value. Suicide offers the clearest example of this. We should take care in saying 'died by suicide' rather than 'commit suicide'. Using the terminology 'commit' implied there is criminality to the act (Volkow et al. 2021). Suicide has not been illegal in the UK since the development of the Suicide Act 1961. Equally, we should not declare suicide attempts as 'successful' or 'unsuccessful' (Volkow et al. 2021).

From Divide to Integration: Where We're Heading

The legacy of division is a hard one to overcome. Whilst some mental health trusts have come together with their general health partners, there remains significant division across many of the services within the UK.

ICS and Mental Health

ICSs offer an opportunity to work across local authorities, NHS, voluntary sectors and others. Indeed, there appears to be a great desire from health leaders to ensure that there is greater integration and to move towards a preventative model. Some ICSs have shown that they are taking steps towards preventing mental health problems and their associated impacts (Mental Health Foundation 2024).

The report *Planning for Prevention—Unlocking the potential of Integrated Care Systems to create a mentally health society* offered some clear recommendations for ICS's, the most pertinent have been discussed further below:

Recommendation 1—Ensure That Plans Are Clear for Public Mental Health
They argue that plans should use clear language, clearly reference to public mental health, and should be based on local need.

Recommendation 2—Better Sharing of Practice
It is important for ICS's and other parties to share the good work they are doing.

Recommendation 3—A Stronger Focus of Minority Communities.
There should be stronger focus on minoritised communities, specifically those for asylum seekers and refugees. There should be clear understanding of the suicidality of these groups.

Recommendation 4—Infrastructure
There should be a creation of public mental health infrastructure which allows central government to address determinants of mental health.

Recommendation 5—More Funding
There should be more money to create infrastructure and to address the gap in mental health spending (Mental Health Foundation 2024).

Community Mental Health Transformation

The Community Mental Health Transformation for adults and older adults with severe mental illness was funded through the NHS Long Term Plan and started in 2019. The model provides further focus on early intervention and assessment and supporting more people to live within their communities. The model advocates for whole-person and whole-population health approaches and working further with primary care networks (NHS England 2023).

Legislative Change—Mental Health Act (2025)

The new Mental Health Act (2025) received Royal Assent in December 2025. A consultation on the Code of Practice is expected in 2026 and will be refreshed most likely in 2027 (NHS Providers 2025a).

Key Learning Points

Mental health affects all elements of our society and communities. We need to expect to see mental health in our service uses, workforce, families and communities.

We need to remember that there is a close, bidirectional relationship between mental and physical health. As an adult or child practitioner, it is important to remember this relationship when assessing and treating service users.

The history of mental health, asylums and the mind-body divide continue to shape the systems we see today. Please remember that much of this separation is historical, and something we continue to wrestle to overcome. There is work we can all do to reduce this divide.

Stigma still impacts the behaviour of service users, such as how and where they seek help. Equally, stigma continues to impact the care and outcomes that service users receive.

Conclusion

This chapter has traced mental health practice from historic foundations to contemporary approaches, showing a profound shift from initialisation to community care. The history of mental health helps explain the separation, stigma and inequity that we continue to fight against in modern mental health practice. We have been able to see how the divide between mental health and health and physical health has been reinforced by funding, attitudes and legislation. Many of the challenges we see in practice today continue to be reinforced by the legacy of separation.

However, throughout the chapter we have seen the relationship between mind and body and potential consequences that not viewing it as such may have. There remain disparities in funding, commissioning and service provision. We must remember the impacts of mortality gap, chronic illness and impact of social determinants in our wider communities.

Understanding the historical, political and structural forces helps us to understand the drivers of mental health care today. Equally, it helps us understand ourselves as practitioners and ensures we can work towards compassionate and equitable person-centred care.

The use of case studies, reflective questions and tasks has helped to ground theory into real-world practice. This has allowed you to apply concepts to your own differing professional contexts and highlights the importance of collaboration and partnership in mental health care.

References

Allin P (2024) A philosophical approach to mental health'. Aust J Gen Pract 53(12 Suppl):S25–S27. https://doi.org/10.31128/AJGP-05-24-7266. Accessed 6 May 2025

Bamert M, Schaffter, Y, Bally F, O'Connor D, Inauen J, (2025) Assessment of stress and its relationship with health behaviour in daily life: a systematic review Health Psychology Review 19(4):906–936. https://doi.org/10.1080/17437199.2025.2534000.

BBC (2025) How a city led a revolution in psychiatric care. BBC News, 19 April. Available at: https://www.bbc.co.uk/news/articles/cvgn594rdr3o. Accessed 15 June 2025

BBC (2026) William says it has taken 'long time to understand my emotions' Available at: https://www.bbc.co.uk/news/articles/cm21d4j26pdo. Accessed 6 June 2026

Bennett JM (2024) The post-cartesian dilemma: reuniting the mind and body through psychoneuroimmunology. Compr Psychoneuroendocrinol 20:100265. https://doi.org/10.1016/j.cpnec.2024.100265

Bentall R, and McKeown M (2024) Critical psychological ideas and practices' in Wright, K. M. and McKeown, M. (eds.) Essentials of Mental Health Nursing. 2nd edn. London: SAGE Publications.

Bourke M, Wang HFW, McNaughton S, Thomas G, Firth J, Trott M, Cairney J (2025) Clusters of healthy lifestyle behaviours are associated with symptoms of depression, anxiety, and psychological distress: a systematic review and meta-analysis of observational studies. Clin Pysychol Rev 118:102585. https://doi.org/10.1016/j.cpr.2025.102585

Care Quality Commission (2018) Under pressure: safely managing increased demand in emergency departments. Care Quality Commission, Newcastle upon Tyne. Available at: https://www.cqc.org.uk/sites/default/files/20180716_underpressure-winterpressures.pdf. Accessed 7 May 2026

Clesse C, Yaqoob MM, Jayakumar S, Bhui K, Carvalho LA (2022) Investigating inflammation in depression in the chronically ill: theoretical model and perspectives. J R Coll Physicians Edinb 52(3):247–252. https://doi.org/10.1177/14782715221115776

Department of Health (2009) Working our way to better mental health: A framework for action. London: The Stationery Office. Available at: https://data.parliament.uk/DepositedPapers/Files/DEP2009-3023/DEP2009-3023.pdf Accessed 22 July 2026

de Vries K, Drury-Ruddlesden J, Gaul C (2019) 'And so I took up residence': the experiences of family members of people with dementia during admission to an acute hospital unit. Dementia 18(1):36–54. https://doi.org/10.1177/1471301216656097

Del Giudice M, Ellis BJ, Shirtcliff EA (2011) The adaptive calibration model of stress responsivity. Neurosci Biobehav Rev 35(7):1562–1592. https://doi.org/10.1016/j.neubiorev.2010.11.007

Del Giudice M, Hinnant JB, Ellis BJ, El-Sheikh M (2012) Adaptive patterns of stress responsivity: a preliminary investigation. Dev Psychol 48(3):775–790. https://doi.org/10.1037/a0026519. Accessed 8 Aug 2025

Deloitte (2024) Poor mental health costs UK employers £51 billion a year for employees. Deloitte UK, 17 May. Available at: https://www.deloitte.com/uk/en/about/press-room/poor-mental-health-costs-uk-employers-51-billion-a-year-for-employees.html. Accessed 7 May 2026

Double D (2024) Psychiatric understandings of mental health. In: Wright KM, McKeown M (eds) Essentials of mental health nursing, 2nd edn. SAGE, London

Eleanor Glanville Institute (n.d.) Madness, gender and class: the Lincoln Lunatic Asylum. Available from: https://eleanorglanvilleinstitute.lincoln.ac.uk/research/research-group-2/the-lincoln-lunatic-asylum/. Accessed 12 December 2025

Garratt R (2024) House of lords reform. Research Briefing CBP-7547. Available at: https://commonslibrary.parliament.uk/research-briefings/cbp-7547/?utm_source=chatgpt.com. Accessed 9 Jun 2026

Ghasemi F, Beversdorf D, Herman K (2024) Stress and stress responses: a narrative literature review from physiological mechanisms to intervention approaches. J Pac Rim Psychol 18:1–20. https://doi.org/10.1177/18344909241289222

Gilburt H, Mallorie S (2024a) Mental health 360. The King's Fund. Available at: https://www.kingsfund.org.uk/insight-and-analysis/long-reads/mental-health-360-workforce. Accessed 15 Jul 2024

Gilburt H, Mallorie S (2024b) Mental health 360: funding and costs. The King's Fund. Available at: https://www.kingsfund.org.uk/insight-and-analysis/long-reads/mental-health-360-funding-costs. Accessed 5 January 2026

Harvard Health (2011) Understanding the stress response. Harvard Health. Available at: https://www.health.harvard.edu/healthy-aging-and-longevity/understanding-the-stress-response. Accessed 12 April 2026

Historic England (2019) From Bethlehem to Bedlam – England's first mental institution. Historicengland.org.uk. Available at: https://historicengland.org.uk/research/inclusive-heritage/disability-history/1050-1485/from-bethlehem-to-bedlam/. Accessed 11 November 2025

Horwitz AV (2012) An overview of sociological perspectives on the definitions, causes, and responses to mental health and illness. In: Horwitz A, Scheid T (eds) A handbook for the study of mental health. Cambridge University Press, Cambridge

Houston R (2019) Asylums: the historical perspective before, during, and after The Lancet Psychiatry, 2019; 7:354–362.

Hulatt I (ed) (2014) Mental health policy for nurses. SAGE Publications Ltd., London

Jayasinghe S (2002) Time to move beyond the mind-body split. BMJ 325:1433–1434. https://doi.org/10.1136/bmj.325.7378.1433

Kantor E, Vuletić G (2023) The relationship between mental health and stress: the moderating role of satisfaction with friendships. Adv Ment Health 22:603–616. https://doi.org/10.1080/18387357.2023.2282046. Accessed 12 Mar 2026.

Kinderman P (2014) Prescription for psychiatry – why we need a whole new approach to mental health and wellbeing. London: Palgrave Macmillan

King's College London (2025) Life expectancy gap for people with severe mental illness is 'hidden health crisis', study finds. Available at: https://www.kcl.ac.uk/news/life-expectancy-gap-for-people-with-severe-mental-illness-is-hidden-health-crisis-study-finds. Accessed 5 June 2026

Liubertiene G, Sloman A, Morris S, Bhavsar V, Clark C, Das-Munshi J, Jenkins R, McManus S, Oram S, Wessely S (2025) Common mental health conditions. In: Morris S, Hill S, Brugha T, McManus S (eds) Adult Psychiatric Morbidity Survey: Survey of Mental Health and Wellbeing, England, 2023/4. NHS England.

McCormack B, McCance T (2006) Development of a framework for person-centred nursing. J Adv Nurs 56(5):472–479

McGrath JJ, Al-Hamzawi A, Alonso J, Altwaijri Y, Andrade LH, Bromet EJ, Bruffaerts R, de Almeida JMC, Chardoul S, Chiu WT, Degenhardt L, Demler OV, Ferry F, Gureje O, Haro JM, Karam EG, Karam G, Khaled SM, Kovess-Masfety V, Magno M, Medina-Mora ME, Moskalewicz J, Navarro-Mateu F, Nishi D, Plana-Ripoll O, Posada-Villa J, Rapsey C, Sampson NA, Stagnaro JC, Stein DJ, Ten Have M, Torres Y, Vladescu C, Woodruff PW, Zarkov Z, Kessler RC (2023) Age of onset and cumulative risk of mental disorders: a cross-national analysis of population surveys from 29 countries. Lancet Psychiatry 10(9):668–681. https://doi.org/10.1016/S2215-0366(23)00193-1

Mental Health Foundation (2019) Why the language we use to describe mental health matters. Available at: https://www.mentalhealth.org.uk/explore-mental-health/blogs/why-language-we-use-describe-mental-health-matters. Accessed 11 December 2025

Mental Health Foundation (2021) Stigma and discrimination. Available at: https://www.mentalhealth.org.uk/explore-mental-health/a-z-topics/stigma-and-discrimination. Accessed 11 December 2025

Mental Health Foundation (2024) Planning for prevention—unlocking the potential of integrated care systems to create a mentally healthy society. Mental Health Foundation, UK. Available at: https://www.mentalhealth.org.uk/sites/default/files/2024-09/MHF%20Integrated%20Care%20Systems%20in%20England%20Report.pdf. Accessed 2 January 2026

Mifsud KR, Reul JMHM (2018) Mineralocorticoid and glucocorticoid receptor-mediated control of genomic responses to stress in the brain. Stress 21(5):389–402. https://doi.org/10.1080/10253890.2018.1456526. Accessed 12 Mar 2026

Miller AC (2006) Jundi-Shapur, bimaristans and the birth of the hospital. J R Soc Med 99(12):624–628

Naylor C et al (2012) Long-term conditions and mental health: the cost of co-morbidities. The King's Fund & Centre for Mental Health, London

NHS (2019) The NHS long term plan. NHS England, London

NHS England (2024) NHS England's NHS mental health services treat record 3.8 million people last year. England.nhs.uk. Available at: https://www.england.nhs.uk/2024/10/englands-nhs-mental-health-services-treat-record-3-8-million-people-last-year/. Accessed 12 Mar 2026

NHS Confederation (2024) Greater than the sum of parts: shared board leadership. Available at: https://www.nhsconfed.org/publications/greater-sum-parts-shared-board-leadership. Accessed 12 Mar 2026

NHS England (2016) The five year forward view for mental Health. NHS England, London

NHS England (2023) Community Mental Health Transformation Programme—partnership with the third sector. Available at: https://www.england.nhs.uk/long-read/nhs-england-community-mental-health-transformation-programme-nhs-partnership-working-with-the-third-sector/. Accessed 12 Mar 2026

NHS England (2025) Improving the physical health of people living with severe mental illness. Available at: https://www.england.nhs.uk/long-read/improving-the-physical-health-of-people-living-with-severe-mental-illness/. Accessed 12 Mar 2026

NHS Providers (2025a) The Mental Health Act 2025: what you need to know. Available at: https://nhsproviders.org/resources/the-mental-health-act-2025-what-you-need-to-know. Accessed 10 October 2025

NHS Providers (2025b) Mental health services: the NHS trust perspective. Available at: https://nhsproviders.org/resources/mental-health-services-the-nhs-trust-perspective. Accessed 14 October 2025

Office for National Statistics (2025) Sickness absence in the UK labour market: 2023 and 2024. Available at: https://www.ons.gov.uk/employmentandlabourmarket/peopleinwork/labourproductivity/articles/sicknessabsenceinthelabourmarket/2023and2024. Accessed 7 May 2026

Ohrnberger J, Fichera E, Sutton M (2017) The relationship between physical and mental health: a mediation analysis. Soc Sci Med 195:42–49

Parliament (UK) (2026) No health without mental health/parity and anti-stigma commitments. Available at: https://www.parliament.uk/business/publications/research/key-issues-parliament-2015/social-change/mental-health-stigma/. Accessed 12 Mar 2026

Pilgrim D, McKeown M (2024) Sociological understandings of mental health. In: Fundamentals of mental health nursing. Sage Publishing, London, pp 217–233

Rössler W (2016) The stigma of mental disorders. Front Public Health 4:29

Science Museum (2018) A Victorian mental asylum. Available at: https://www.sciencemuseum.org.uk/objects-and-stories/medicine/victorian-mental-asylum Accessed 10 September 2025

Selby, H. (2020) 'Continuity and Change in British Public Service Television's Engagement with Mental Health', VIEW Journal of European Television History and Culture, 9(18):126–140. Available at: https://doi.org/10.18146/view.226

Sidi L (2021) After the madhouses: the emotional politics of psychiatry and community care in the UK tabloid press 1980–1995. Med Humanit 48(4):medhum-2020-012117. https://doi.org/10.1136/medhum-2020-012117

Suicide Act (1961) (9 and 10 Eliz. 2, c.60). HMSO, London
The Health Foundation (2024) Health conditions among working-age adults Available at: https://www.health.org.uk/resources-and-toolkits/data-tools/evidence-hub/health-conditions-among-working-age-people. Accessed 9 May 2026
Thibaut F (2018) The mind-body cartesian dualism and psychiatry. Dialogues Clin Neurosci 20(1):3–3. https://doi.org/10.31887/DCNS.2018.20.1/fthibaut. Accessed 14 Mar 2025
Thornton T (2024) Philosophical understanding of mental health. In: Essentials of mental Health nursing, 2nd edn. SAGE, London. ISBN 9781529733044. Accessed 14 Mar 2025
Turner J, Hayward R, Angel K, Fulford B, Hall J, Millard C, Thomson M (2015) The history of mental health services in modern England: practitioner memories and the direction of future research. Med Hist 59(4):599–624. https://doi.org/10.1017/mdh.2015.48
Ventriglio A, Bhugra D (2015) Mind–body dualism and integration in psychiatry. Int Rev Psychiatry 27(5):463–465
Volkow ND, Gordon JA, Koob GF (2021) Choosing appropriate language to reduce the stigma around mental illness and substance use disorders. Neuropsychopharmacology 46(13):2230–2232. https://doi.org/10.1038/s41386-021-01069-4
WHO (2022) Suicide worldwide in 2021. World Health Organization, Geneva
WHO (2025) Global mental health estimates. World Health Organization, Geneva
Wickens C (2022) Provider collaboratives: explaining their role in system working. The King's Fund. Available at: https://www.kingsfund.org.uk/insight-and-analysis/long-reads/provider-collaboratives. Accessed 16 October 2026
Wilson H, Finch D (2021) Unemployment and mental health: why both require action for our COVID-19 recovery. The Health Foundation, London. Available at: https://www.health.org.uk/sites/default/files/2021-04/2021%20-%20Unemployment%20and%20mental%20health.pdf. Accessed 7 May 2026
Yin Y, Ju T, Zeng D, Duan F, Zhu Y, Liu J, Li Y, Lu W (2024) 'Inflamed' depression: a review of the interactions between depression and inflammation and current anti-inflammatory strategies for depression. Pharmacol Res 207:107322. https://doi.org/10.1016/j.phrs.2024.107322. Accessed 8 March 2026
Zhao Y, Yang L, Sahakian BJ, Langley C, Zhang W, Kuo K, Li Z, Gan Y, Li Y, Zhao Y, Yu J, Feng J, Cheng W (2023) The brain structure, immunometabolic and genetic mechanisms underlying the association between lifestyle and depression. Nat Ment Health 1(10):736–750. https://doi.org/10.1038/s44220-023-00120-1.
Zunszain PA, Hepgul N, Pariante CM (2012) Inflammation and depression. In: Cowen P, Sharp T, Lau J (eds) Behavioral neurobiology of depression and its treatment. Current topics in behavioral neurosciences, vol 14. Springer, Berlin, Heidelberg. https://doi.org/10.1007/7854_2012_211

Person-Centred Care

Reflective Questions
What does meaningful service user involvement mean to you?
What did person-centred care mean to you?
When do you feel confident, or uncertain, communicating with someone in distress, and what shapes that feeling?

We should recognise that person-centred care is mentioned in many of our professional codes of conduct and handbooks, such as:

> Demonstrate self-awareness with compassionate and inspirational leadership with interprofessional teams to influence practice for effective, holistic, person-centred care. (NMC 2018)

> As a health and care professional, you must promote and protect the interests of service users and carers. What we mean by this is:
>
> - Treating service users and carers with respect.
> - Making sure you have consent.
> - Challenging discrimination.
> - Maintaining appropriate boundaries. (HCPC 2014)

What Is Person-Centred Care?

Person-centred care has become increasingly prominent in health and social care in the recent decades (Lombard 2024). Whilst the term, person-centred care, is now largely used, you may have seen a range of terminology in literature to refer to similar principles such as patient-centred care, personalisation, mutuality and relationship-centred care (The Health Foundation 2016).

R. Bage, *Mental Health Skills for Adult Nurses & Non-Specialist Healthcare Workers*, https://doi.org/10.1007/978-3-032-32835-9_2

The VIPS definition of person-centred came in 2004 and was in response to policy definitions in the UK which confused person-centred care and individualised care (Brooker and Latham 2016). The VIPS definition consisted of four central elements (Brooker 2003), which is shown in Table 1 (Brooker and Latham 2016).

VIPS was later simplified to the following:

V—A value based that asserts the absolute value of all human lives regardless of age or cognitive ability.
I—An individualised approach, recognising uniqueness.

Table 1 VIPS definition of person-centred care

Person-centred care and definition	Key indicators
Valuing people Valuing people who live with dementia and those who care for them—promoting rights and entitlements regardless of age or cognitive ability and rooting out discriminatory practice	Vision Human resources Management ethos Training and staff development Service environments Quality assurance
Individual lives This is about recognising that all people are difference. Ensuring that people are recognised as individuals, appreciating that all people have a unique history and personality, physical and psychological strengths and needs, and social and economic resources and that those will affect their response to dementia	Care and support plans Regular reviews Personal possessions Individual preferences Life stories Activity and occupation
Personal perspectives This focusses on looking at the world from the perspective of the person living with dementia. It focusses on recognising that each person's experiences have their own psychological validity, that people act from this perspective and empathy with this perspective has its own therapeutic potential	Communication Empathy and acceptable risk Environment Physical health Challenging behaviour as communication Advocacy
Social environment This looks at providing a social environment that supports psychological needs: providing a supportive social environment requires the recognition that all human life is grounded in relationships and that people living with dementia need an enriched social environment that compensates for their impairment and allows opportunities for personal growth	Inclusion Respect Warmth Validation Enabling Part of the community Relationships

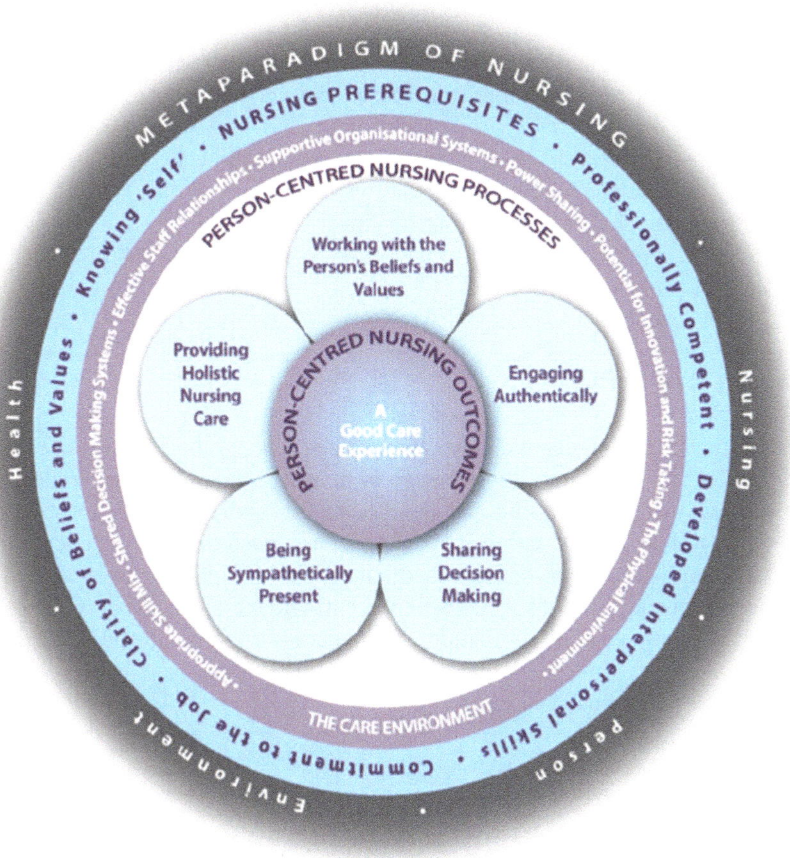

Fig. 1 Person-centred nursing framework

P—Understanding the worlds from the perspective of the person identified as needing support.

S—Providing a social environment that supports psychological needs (Brooker and Latham 2016).

The parts of the VIPS definition are titled the 'elements of person-centred care', appreciating that all of the elements exist independently of each other. You may also see it expressed as PCC (person-centred care) = V + I + P + S (Brooker and Latham 2016).

McCormack and McCance (2025) developed a framework, seen in Fig. 1 and used with agreement from the authors, for person-centred care in 2006. The framework comprises four constructs—prerequisites, care environment, person-centred processes and expected outcomes. The framework suggests that account must be taken of the prerequisites and the care environment that are required for effective care.

The Health Foundation (2016) has also produced their own principles of person-centred care. They consider four principles of person-centred care:

1. Affording people to have dignity, compassion and respect
2. Offering coordinated care, support or treatment
3. Offering personal care, support or treatment
4. Supporting people to recognise and develop strengths and abilities to live an independent and fulfilling life.

The History of PCC

The origins of person-centred care can be traced to a psychotherapist, Carl Rogers (1952). Rogers was one of the pioneers of humanistic psychology, an idea which moved away from the traditional psychoanalysis and behaviourism approaches (Yao and Kabir 2023; Joseph 2014). Rogers introduced the idea of 'client-centred therapy' amongst mental health practitioners, an idea that focussed on building warm and trusting relationships between clients and therapists (Rogers 1952).

Rogers identified that six conditions were necessary for therapeutic change:

1. Therapist–client psychological contact.
2. Client incongruence.
3. Therapist congruence.
4. Therapist unconditional positive regard.
5. Therapist empathetic understanding.
6. Client perception (Yao and Kabir 2023).

Rogers also went on to define three attitudes needed by therapists that are key to person-centred therapies:

Accurate Empathy

This focusses on ideas such as active listening and paying key focus on the client's feelings and thoughts. One helpful technique for this is reflection, focussing on paraphrasing and/or summarising of the feeling behind what is said. This allows space for the clients to process their feelings after hearing them restated by someone else (Yao and Kabir 2023).

Congruence

The therapist conveys feelings and thoughts that genuinely relate to the client. The therapist should be genuinely himself. Therapists may share emotional reactions with their clients but do not share their personal problems (Yao and Kabir 2023).

Unconditional Positive Regard

This is when a therapist creates a warm environment that conveys to clients that they are accepted unconditionally. There should be no judgement, approval or disapproval, no matter how unconventional the client's views may be. This allows opportunities for the clients to drop natural defences, allowing them to freely express feelings (Yao and Kabir 2023).

George Engel's biopsychosocial model was developed in the 1980s and is also a key model in the development of person-centred care. Designed to be a new way of thinking, it moved away from the biomedical models of health, which he considered reductionist, to a new scientific model which focussed on the relationship between mind–body (Card 2022).

Professor Kitwood was an English Academic who was key in the development of person-centred approaches in dementia care, during the 1990s, about 10 years after the development of the biopsychosocial model. Kitwood was thought to use the term 'person-centred' care in regard to be bringing ideas and ways of working together regards lived experiences, communication and relationships (Brooker and Latham 2016). Kitwood's ideas built on Roger's psychotherapy work 30 years previously. Kitwood sadly died in 1998, just after the publication of *Dementia Reconsidered,* which was probably his best-known title.

Kitwood focussed on key themes such as personhood, malignant social psychology, psychological needs of people with dementia and positive people work (Kelly et al. 2023). Kitwood defines personhood as 'a standing or status that is bestowed upon one human being by others, in the context of relationship and social being. It implies recognition, respect, and trust' (Kitwood 1997). Personhood is essentially what we want to protect when delivering person-centred care.

Person-Centred Care and Mental Health

Mental health practice through the history has bounced between humane and oppressive. Historically, it has focussed very much on diagnoses and classification, rather than backgrounds, cultures and trauma. With the power for service users to be detained against their will, there remain conflicts between professionals and service users and the conflict between personal and public good (Boardman and Dave 2020).

Boardman and Dave (2020) suggested five considerations for mental health psychiatrist and person-centred approaches which can relate to the wider field of health care. These are summarised in Table 2 (Boardman and Dave 2020).

Table 2 Five considerations of mental health and person-centred approaches

Consideration	Details
Rights	Mental health practice can involve restricting personal freedom Importance for clinicians to have knowledge of human rights and legislation Idea of proportionality
Relationships	Become recovery-focussed Understand service user history, strengths, goals, social circumstances, activities, beliefs, spirituality, values, etc. Understand what the service user would like to achieve in their life Codesigning of plans with professionals
Importance to clinicians	Understand that clinicians are people too—and wellbeing of practitioners has a direct impact on care.
Values	Collaborative resolution of conflicts between stakeholders (e.g. nurse/doctor/service user) All professionals have similar guidelines
Training	Embedding person-centred care approaches into training and assessment

A systematic review by Khosravi et al. (2024) identified six key themes of person-centredness in mental health services:

Education

Khosravi et al. (2024) found that the provision of education and information to service users was key in the person-centred delivery of care. This included elements such as information about their mental health problem, treatment and psychoeducation.

Involvement and Cooperation

Person-centred care in mental health focusses on engaging and collaborating with families, service users and friends. Khosravi et al. (2024) found that this collaboration was important to ensure that service users had the opportunity to exercise autonomy and dignity.

Access

Khosvari et al. (2024) found that person-centred care requires timely access to services, with prompt access to care demonstrating real benefits.

Effectiveness and Safety

Khosvari et al. (2024) found that the safety and effectiveness of certain aspects of care were important in the delivery of person-centred care. These factors included psychopharmacology and medication delivery, psychological care, environment of care delivery and continuity of care (Khosvari et al. 2024).

Ethics

Ensuring that practitioners are respectful and offer dignity for service users is important for person-centred care. Equally, it is important to ensure that people's personal data is protected is a major pillar for person-centred care in mental health services (Khosvari et al. 2024).

Health and Wellbeing

Ensuring that practitioners consider emotional, psychological, social, behavioural, interpersonal, physical and personal aspects of life is considered important in the delivery of person-centred care.

Case Study

Amira has a diagnosis of bipolar disorder and is prescribed quetiapine which she takes daily. Her last secondary care review was 10 months ago when she asked to be discharged to her GP. She said at this appointment that staying with Secondary Care made her feel 'unwell'. She lives alone and works part-time in the local Students Union as a graphic designer. Amira has been off sick for the last 10 days. Within these 10 days, she has presented twice to the pharmacist in this period with 'racing thoughts' and 'poor sleep'.

Amira has attended a same-day appointment for insomnia, which was made by her sister. She is very animated in the waiting room, pacing and talking loudly on her phone. She reports that she is sleeping for 3 hours a night as she is feeling very productive and taking on lots of freelance work. She reports that she is planning to set up her own business and plans to go and buy all the new technology and digital art materials that she needs after this appointment and before her 'inspiration' goes. Amira tells you that life is going so well that she has stopped taking her quetiapine as it is making her feel 'foggy'.

Questions

What are your concerns when supporting Amira?

How do you balance Amira's autonomy and creativity whilst also discussing and assessing her risk?

How can you ensure you are communicating with Amira in a person-centred way throughout the consultation?

Personal Recovery

There are several models used within mental health services that focus in on recovery and person-centred care. Over recent times, the concepts of recovery and person-centredness have become popular within policy, practice and research (Hummelvol et al. 2015). Recovery, like person-centred care, looks at ideas such as finding meaning and control, with support for decision-making and partnerships (Hummelvol et al. 2015). Personal recovery can be considered a very individualised process in changing attitudes, values, feelings, goals, skills or roles to support living a satisfying, hopeful and contributing life without limitations caused by illness or ill health (Anthony 1993). Other definitions include:

> Overcoming the effects of being a service user in mental health care and regaining some degree of control over your own life. (Davidson et al. 2005)

> A way of living a satisfying, fulfilling and hopeful live even with the limitations of ill health. (Anthony 1993)

Whilst personal recovery focuses on areas such as attitudes, values, feelings, goals, meaning and purpose, clinical recovery should be seen as quite different. Personal recovery and clinical recovery have been found to be only modestly related to each other (Yu et al. 2022). Clinical recovery can be defined as the reduction of symptoms and return to a 'normal' level of functioning (Van Eck et al. 2018). Slade (2009) considers that clinical recovery has four factors:

1. It is an outcome or a state.
2. It is observable, and this is objective.
3. It is rated by the professional, not the service user.
4. The definition of recovery is invariant across service users and groups.

Liberman et al. (2002) offer a different example of recovery based on service users with schizophrenia over a period of two consecutive years:

1. Symptom remission.
2. Full- or part-time involvement in school or work environment.
3. Independent living without supervision.
4. Not fully dependent on financial support.
5. Have friends to share activities with.

In mental health, there is argument that treatment needs to focus on interventions that target both clinical and personal recovery (Austin et al. 2022).

Case Study

Concerns for Amira relate to her current mental state and her lack of insight into her current mental health. There is also urgency with this because she is talking about going to spend money this afternoon on something that she may later regret. This spending money is a key indicator for a bipolar relapse.

When assessing autonomy and creativity with Amira, you would want to be exploring her current plan for her business and how reasonable and practical these plans are. You will want to be ensuring that she is making these decisions with full capacity and insight into her decision-making. You also need to be conscious that Amira has stopped taking her medication.

The first stage in this is developing a therapeutic relationship with Amria, focussing on open body language and conversation. You will want to be exploring your concerns and worries with Amira in a very open way, if she can manage this openness. However, in Amira's case, this may risk her becoming agitated.

In Amira's case, I would be escalating this immediately to mental health services and specialists. This is due to her escalating behaviour, lack of medication adherence and agitated behaviour in the waiting room. It may be that Amira needs hospitalisation for a period of stabilisation.

Reflective Question

What happened when you imposed a clinical goal that clashed with a person's recovery goal? What happened?

The Recovery Model was primarily led from consumer groups who pushed for services to adopt the model (Jacobson and Greenley 2001). The model shows a significant shift in the use of the word 'recovery', moving from the idea of recovery = fixed, to an idea where you can live a meaningful life even whilst suffering from a mental illness (Cruwys et al. 2020). The recovery model has four key areas of focus: hope, healing, empowerment and connection and is shown in Table 3 (adapted from Jacobson and Greenley 2001).

The Conceptual framework for personal recovery in mental health (CHIME) was published in 2001 by Leamy et al. (2011). This model has become dominant in current mental health practice (Hurst et al. 2025). This conceptual framework has five key recovery processes and is shown in Fig. 2 (Omundo et al. 2025).

CHIME has been seen to be used in multiple cultures (e.g. Apostopoulou et al. 2020; Brijnath 2015). One criticism of the CHIME model is that it may not provide the depth required. A systematic review completed in 2016 found evidence that expansion of themes within CHIME may be needed. These new themes included difficulties, an idea where area of struggle is included, to avoid the potential misconception that those struggling with recovery are 'not trying hard enough' (Stuart et al. 2017). Some difficulties we may see may be financial or interpersonal, and individuals may not have full control of making these changes.

Table 3 Recovery model

Hope	At a basic level, this is around a person's belief that recovery is possible. Hope looks at ideas such as recognising and accepting the problem, committing to change, strength-based thinking, focuses and positives rather than weaknesses, celebrating small successes and being optimism
Healing	The recovery model looks at the idea that healing has two main components, defining a self apart from illness, and control
Empowerment	Empowerment has three main ideas—autonomy, courage and responsibility. Autonomy looks at the ideas of knowledge, self-confidence and the availability of meaningful choices. Courage looks at the willingness to take risks, to speak independently and to step outside of normal routines. With the recovery model considers that service users should have increased responsibility for themselves. These responsibilities include developing goals, working with providers and engaging in self-care
Connection	Connection looks at recovery as a social process. It considers the importance of joining the social world, to forge connections and to find roles in the world

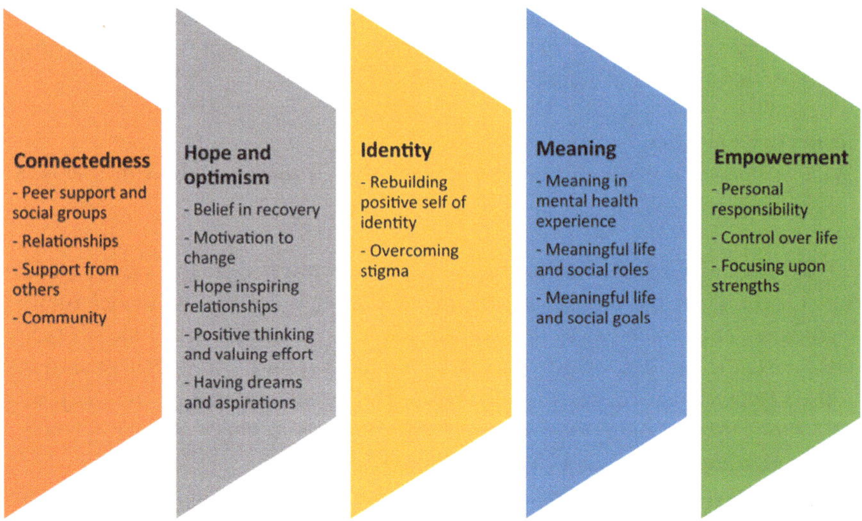

Fig. 2 CHIME model (Omundo et al. 2025 used under Creative Commons Licence). (From Science Direct, Elsevier, https://doi.org/10.1108/JMHTEP-05-2024-0052, licenced under CC-BY 4.0)

A further theme not included in the model could be acceptance. Ideas within this could be ideas such as accepting limitations, having patience and learning to focus on the present (Stuart et al. 2017). The final theme discussed in the systematic review looks at the desire to return to normality (Stuart et al. 2017).

Patient Involvement

Coproduction of mental health services, and services on the whole, should now be seen as gold standard (Stanyon et al. 2024). Recent legislation and policy such as *The Five-Year Forward View for Mental Health* ((NHS England 2016) and *NHS Long Term Plan* (NHS 2019) highlighted the importance of service user involvement and shared decision-maker. However, we will all have experienced times when service user involvement has not worked well. The Board Meetings, where the service user chair was introduced to ensure decision-makers thought about the service user, without a service user being actually invited is a specific one that will live long in the memory.

Equally, nursing regulators in the UK require service users to be involved in the development, delivery and evaluation of nursing curriculum (Terry and Garner 2024).

There are significant benefits of patient involvement within mental health services, and these have been discussed below (Terry and Garner 2024):

Experts in Experiences

Service users have the best knowledge of their mental health, experience and life. Nobody else could possibly have the same level of knowledge or experience about their mental health problems and journey in mental health services.

Different Strategies

Many service users will have developed their own list of coping mechanisms which help them manage their own mental health conditions. Many service users have learnt to predict and manage their own mental health. This is information that is useful for professionals.

Perspectives

Service users will have their own perspectives on treatment and care, and this will often allow practitioners and services to reflect on the services they are delivering. This open dialogue can help practitioners and services be critical about what they are delivering and then deliver change.

Therapeutic

Some service users will get a real benefit from engaging and involving with services and service change and in turn improve confidence and self-esteem. It can also be a beneficial experience for professionals involved.

Patient Experts and Lived Experience

Reflective Questions
What has been your experience to do with experts by experience?
Does your services have lived experience roles? Why?

The term 'expert patient' gained popularity after being used by the chief medical officer in the early 2000s.. Early introduction was mixed, with term frequently being criticised by medical professionals.

However, this change was not a quick one. The biomedical model of medicine has put the doctor, or clinician, as the boss. However, in the early millennium we started to see this change. The public became better educated, by a variety of choice and media, and the public became better educated of their rights. There was also a change to not be a passive receiver of goods or services but instead became consumers with the expectation of good-quality service with a right to complain (Kennedy 2003).

We have also moved towards self-management. Self-management is an approach aimed at improving a service users' quality of life through increased self-efficacy (Franek 2013). Self-management does however make some assumptions about our service users. Integral to the idea is that service users want to be informed, activated and expert service users, with an idea that they can overcome structural determinants which exist in social concepts (Bodenheimer et al. 2002).

Peer support workers have occurred across history, with the idea that service users come together to provide informal support (Faulkner and Basset 2012). Lived experience, or peer workers, are now recognised across mental health services (Robinson and Isaacs 2025). Workers with individuals' lived experiences of mental health difficulties were present in many recent reports including the 5 Year Forward View for Mental Health and the NHS Long Term Plan (2019).

The 'Competence Framework for Mental Health Peer support workers' was developed by Health Education England (2020). This sets out nine domains for peer support workers:

1. Understanding the values of peer support and the principles that underpin them.
2. Knowledge for peer support works.
3. Core relational skills.
4. Supporting people as a peer support worker.
5. Working with teams and promoting people's rights.
6. Self-care and support.
7. Meta-competencies for peer support workers.
8. Optional Skills: Using psychological approaches to support personal recovery.
9. Competencies for organisations supporting the peer worker role.

Criticism of this framework has been significant, however. The National Survivor User Network (NSUN) was critical due to not drawing on shared understandings of peer support and its 'prescriptive and clinical' nature. They also highlighted the lack of peer support workers, people with lived experience or leading researchers in developing the framework (NSUN 2020).

Some research has been completed into the impact of peer support workers in practice. A systematic review and meta-analysis found that the involvement of one-to-one peer support in mental health services may positively impact psychosocial outcomes (White et al. 2020).

Shared Decision-Making (SDM) in Practice

Shared decision-making in mental health practice looks at clinicians and service users working together to make decisions in practice (Slade 2017). It is a key approach to promoting person-centred care and recovery practices within healthcare settings (Gurtner et al. 2024). A common definition is as follows:

'a process in which clinicians and service users work together to select tests, treatments, management or support packages, based on clinical evidence and the patient's informed preferences; it involves the provision of evidence-based information about options, outcomes and uncertainties, together with decision support counselling and a system for recording and implementing service users' informed preferences' (Coulter and Collins 2011).

Relational Communication is key to the idea of shared decision-making (Kunneman et al. 2019). There has been significant drive for shared decision-making to become the norm within the UK health system. Equally, professional regulatory bodies across the health system consider shared decision-making to be an important ethical commitment (Coulter and Collins 2011). Shared decision-making was included in the NHS Long Term Plan's commitment to make personalised care the norm (NHS England).

NICE (2026) have identified a number of benefits for shared decision-making in practice:

- It allows an open discussion about sharing information. This helps to make sure people have an understanding of benefits and harms of different options.
- It empowers people to make decisions about the treatment and care that is right for them. For some people, choosing no treatment is the right choice.
- It allows people to consider how involved they want to be in decision-making regarding their care.

Shared decision-making in mental health looks much the same as in other healthcare settings. Examples could include pharmaceutical change, whether to undergo a medical procedure, or whether to complete a diagnostic test (Slade 2017). Decision-making in the community could be seen as much wide ranging, in both adult and mental health fields, focussing on treatments, social and financial factors (Freidl et al. 2016). Shared decision-making is promoted in mental health systems and is consistently in policy from around the world (Slade 2017). However, there are known barriers to shared decision-making in mental health practice. For example, some service users will not want to be involved in their care planning decisions. As professionals, it is important that we recognise this and respect their wishes. However, we also need to ensure that we consider that this might change. In mental health, fluctuating levels of motivation, energy and activity may impact people's willingness to engage in decisions about their care. You may find that people want to become more involved as their health and mental health improve (Terry and Garner 2024).

Advanced Directives

Some service users within mental health services will have advance directives or decisions (Terry and Garner 2024). Advance directives are decisions that are written statements that set down your preferences, wishes, beliefs and values regarding any future care. This could include elements about religion, spirituality, where you would like to be care for and how you like to do things (such as what you eat or how to clean yourself). If may also include practical steps such as who would look after your cat if you were to have to go into hospital (NHS 2025). Even if service users are detained under the Mental Health Act (1983), professionals must consider wishes of the service user wherever possible.

If you are caring for somebody who is unable to verbalise their wishes, it is important to ascertain whether they have an advanced directive. They may have shared copies with mental health professionals, social services or a relative or advocate.

Decision Aids

Patient decisions aids vary in type. They could be a page-long document outlining their current choices, to interactive videos or filmed content. Decisions aids differ from traditional patient literature as they do not tell people what to do (The King's Fund 2011). They may contain:

- A description of the illness and/or symptoms.
- Likely prognosis (with and without intervention).
- Treatment or self-management available.
- Outcome probabilities.
- What is known from the evidence.
- Whether there are any gaps in knowledge.
- Illustrations to help people understand experiences.
- A means of helping clarify preferences or rankings.
- Further reading and references (The Kings Fund 2011).

There are a number of decisions aids available. A Cochrane review in 2009 (O'Connor et al. 2001) reviewed 55 studies and found that patient decision aids led to greater knowledge, a better understanding of risk, greater participation in decision-making and no risk in anxiety.

NICE (2026) have developed several patient decision aids which are there to support people in deciding on healthcare options. These offer an evidence-based tool to support decision-making in practice.

Measuring What Matters

One challenge with person-centred care is that it can focus too much on processes and outcomes. This can become challenging when the outcomes are on a narrow focus on measurable health status changes. In most cases, person-centred care cannot compete with interventions which are more directly linked to health status outcomes (Entwistle and Watt 2013). We all know that some of the biggest successes in health care are not necessarily measurable but are the ones that stick with you throughout your career. In my own practice, ensuring that two people with early dementia and a learning disability were supported to stay together was something that mattered, because it was delivering that person-centred care.

A study in 2018 found that five out of twelve countries surveyed regularly collected patient-reported outcome measures (PROMs) and patient-reported experience measures (PREMs) on a regular basis (de Bienassis et al. 2021).

PROMs are questionnaires completed by service users. PROMs are used by service users and practitioners to help understand and measure health and wellbeing before, during and after support, care and treatment.

PROM's can be helpful for:

- Allowing service users space to express themselves.
- Clarify how people are feeling.
- Allow people to feel understood.
- Focus on the important bits.
- Demonstrate they are making progress.
- Offer personalised and appropriate care.

PROMs used commonly in mental health outpatient care include the DIALOG scale, Goal-Based Outcomes tool and Recovering Quality of Life Scale.

Patient-reported experience measures (PREMs) are a measure of patient experience. PREMs are typically gathered through survey or questionnaire and record an experience of health care. This includes elements such as staff communication, how they were treated or communication with services (de Bienassis et al. 2021).

De Bienassis et al. (2021) identified some key questions to consider before the use of PROMs and PREMs in mental health care:

- Are the instruments scientifically acceptable? (e.g. are they reliable and valid?)
- Is a generic- or condition-specific PROM/PREM most appropriate?

- Have service users been involved in stages of identifying and choosing what measures are meaningful?
- Can the PROM/PREMs be integrated into the existing systems of care?
- Is the burden of data collection on service users acceptable given the information that will be generated?
- Will information generate lead to actionable results?

There needs to be balance in their use in mental health services. PROMs are often used dually as tools to measure change in outcomes and screening tools to inform mental health condition diagnosis (de Bienassis et al. 2021). PROMs can help healthcare assess whether treatments deliver good value for money and can track population health trends overtime. However, there remain issues in accurate completion if questionnaires are too long or do not use person-centred language. Equally, PROMs and PREMs need the infrastructure and security/privacy behind them for service users to complete (Benson 2025).

Barriers and Enablers to Person-Centred Care

Reflective Questions

What are the barriers or enablers for delivering person-centred care in your work environment?

Do you have any concerns about delivering person-centred care in the field of mental health?

Communication

One of the challenges of person-centred care is poor communication skills. Communication helps provide a relationship with a service user and benefit person-centred outcomes (Sharkiya 2023). However, communication is often impacted by barriers such as institutional, environmental and personal/behavioural barriers. As a professional, one of our roles is to highlight these challenges (Kwame and Petrucka 2021).

Kwame and Petrucka (2021) proposed a model, see Fig. 3, looking at person-centred care and communication which helps to orientate healthcare professionals in care and communication contents. They describe that task-centred communication, at the lowest level of the PC4 model, is around tasks that are done as fast as possible with little to no communication. Some of the motivations for task-centred communication is time limitation, high workload and staff shortages. Process-centred communication is in the middle of the continuum and could slip between task-centred or person-centred communication. Process-centred communicators try to know their service users as they perform care tasks. They may not encourage service users to express their thoughts, but they do recognise service users as individuals. This involved more informative and less authoritative communication. The

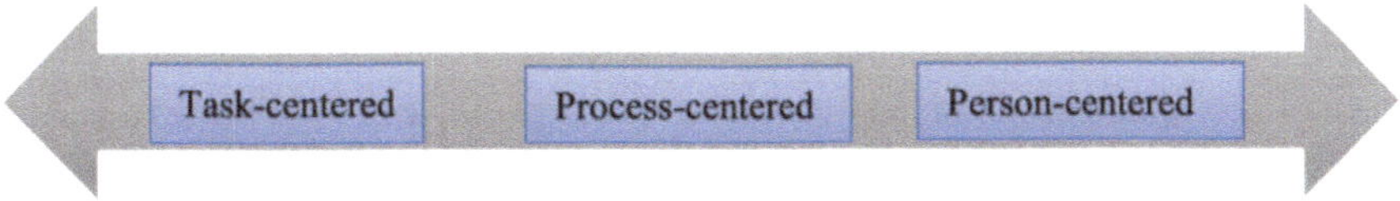

Fig. 3 Person-centred care and communication continuum (PC4 Model). (From BMC Nursing, Springer, https://doi.org/10.1186/s12912-021-00684-2, licenced under CC-BY 4.0)

highest part of the PC4 model looks at where person-centred care is achieved. People are treated as unique people with specific care needs and collaborators in their care. This is at the point of when people create meaningful relationships with service users. This stage of the process requires people to show active listening, genuine interest, respect and warmth (Kwame and Petrucka 2021).

In A + E services, person-centred care to mental health service users may not be delivered due to some of these barriers. It is often hectic, changeable and unpredictable. This makes it a challenging environment for the service users and for the staff. It simply often is not the easiest environment to ensure you are considering person-centred communication.

Task

Using the PC4 model as a basis, consider your communication to your service users on the last day you worked.

Where would you place your communication?
Would you have more communication in the task-centred or person-centred categories?
Why do you think this might be?
Do you have barriers to communicating in a person-centred way?

Family and Carers

One of the challenges with delivering person-centred care is when there are differences of opinions between families and/or carers. It can be hard as professionals to balance when families or carers have different expectations or priorities (Price 2020). In practice, we know that establishing that all people who are involved in the care of a service user to be happy can be challenging, and at some points, not everybody will be happy. However, it is important we try and cater for all the needs and support goals that are needed.

Professional Relationships

One of the challenges in mental health has been the impact of the professional and the relationship with the professionals involved. A thematic analysis looking into patient-centredness in mental health services found that service user decision-making is impacted by relationships with their psychologists (Khosravi et al. 2024). However, equally the power balance is often still inclined heavily towards professionals, with a 2016 paper reporting that only 60% of service users' feelings they are involved in their own care decisions (Fisher 2016). Equally, there are studies that suggest that some psychiatrists can overrate their own performance and ability to work as part of a team. This will no doubt also be present in other professionals working with people who have mental ill health.

Key Learning Points

Please remember that a person is always more important than a diagnosis. It is important we remember what makes a person unique. Please always remember to ask preferences and values, rather than assumptions based on what we think we know about a diagnosis.

We should all be using shared decision-making as the basis of our practice whenever possible. This means people get to help make decisions about their own care. We should also make sure that a person's important people are also involved whenever this is possible—such as family and carers.

We should never make assumptions about recovery—personal recovery and clinical recovery mean very different things. We should always make sure that we understand what a service user wants.

We should make sure that when service users are unwell, we continue to respect consent, dignity, boundaries and non-discriminatory practice.

Conclusion

Person-centred care remains an evolving and influential aspect of mental health practice, and there is little indication that this will change in near future. Models of person-centred care and recovery discussed throughout this chapter have helped demonstrate that ideas are not just goals but can be achievable in contemporary practice. When applied with thought and support, person-centred care can offer a framework for care that is responsive and effective for our service users.

Within this chapter, we have had the opportunity to reflect why person-centred care remains complex within everyday practice. Discussions around organisational and communication barriers, power imbalances and professional competence have helped us understood why we may not consistently see person-centred care in practice. However, despite these challenges, we can see that ideas around collaboration, engagement and recognition of experiences improve the effectiveness and quality of care. By acknowledging these challenges, we can start to address them rather than accepting as unavoidable barriers.

Person-centred care is grounded in collaboration, engagement and recognition of lived experience. When service users are listened to, and involved in decision-making, their care becomes more recovery-focussed and relevant. Person-centred care helps to support stronger therapeutic relationships and improve trust.

What is clear is that this is not just a new policy, performance target or outcome. This requires us to completely shift our way of thinking. For some of us, that shift is hugely away from what we were traditional models and practices we were taught or witnessed in our early practice. This change can be challenging. However, this new approach allows us to work in a way that work bests for our service users and keeps them at the core of what we are doing.

References

Anthony WA (1993) Recovery from mental illness: the guiding vision of the mental health service system in the 1990s. Psychosoc Rehabil J 16(4):11–23

Apostolopoulou A, Stylianidi, S, Issari P, Chondros P, Alexiadou A, Belekou P, Giannou C, Karali EK, Foi V, Tzaferou F (2020) Experiences of Recovery in EPAPSY's Community Residential Facilities and the Five CHIME Concepts: A Qualitative Inquiry, Frontiers in Psychiatry, 11, Article 24. Available at: https://doi.org/10.3389/fpsyt.2020.00024

Austin SF, Hjorthøj C, Baagland H, Simonsen E, Dam J (2022) Investigating personal and clinical recovery processes in people with first episode psychosis. Early Interv Psychiatry 16(10):1102–1111. https://doi.org/10.1111/eip.13258. Accessed 7 Feb 2026

Benson T, (2025) Why health services should use generic PROMs and PREMs' BMJ Open Quality, 14(4), e003435. Available at: doi: 10.1136/bmjoq-2025-003435.

de Bienassis K, Kristensen S, Hewlett E, Roe D, Mainz J, Klazinga N (2021) Patient-reported indicators in mental health care: towards international standards among members of the OECD. Int J Qual Health Care 33(1):ii7–ii12. https://doi.org/10.1093/intqhc/mzab020. Accessed 9 Feb 2025

Boardman J, Dave S (2020) Person-centred care and psychiatry: some key perspectives. BJPsych Int 17(3):1–4. https://doi.org/10.1192/bji.2020.21. Accessed 9 Feb 2025

Bodenheimer T, Lorig K, Holman H, Grumbach K (2002) Patient self-management of chronic disease. JAMA 288(19):2469–2475

Brijnath, B. (2015) Applying the CHIME recovery framework in two culturally diverse Australian communities: Qualitative results International Journal of Social Psychiatry, 61(7):660–667. Available at: https://doi.org/10.1177/0020764015573084

Brooker D, Latham I (2016) Person-centred dementia care: making services better with the VIPS framework. Jessica Kingsley, London

Brooker D (2003) 'What is person-centred care in dementia?', Reviews in Clinical Gerontology 13(3):215–222. https://doi.org/10.1017/S095925980400108X. Accessed 8 February 2025.

Card A (2023) The biopsychosociotechnical model: a systems-based framework for human-centered health improvement, Health Systems, 12(4):387–407. Available at: https://doi.org/10.1080/20476965.2022.2029584. Accessed 8 January 2025

Coulter A, Collins A (2011) Making shared decision-making a reality. The King's Fund. Accessed 8 May 2025

Cruwys T, Stewart B, Buckley L, Gumley J, Scholz B (2020) The recovery model in chronic mental health: A community-based investigation of social identity processes, Psychiatry Research, 291, Article 113241. Available at: https://doi.org/10.1016/j.psychres.2020.113241.

Davidson L, O'Connell MJ, Tondora J, Lawless M, Evans AC (2005) Recovery in serious mental illness: a new wine or just a new bottle? Prof Psychol Res Pract 36(5):480–487. https://doi.org/10.1037/0735-7028.36.5.480
HEE (2020) Competence framework for mental health peer support workers. Health Education England, London. https://www.health.org.uk/sites/default/files/PersonCentredCareMadeSimple.pdf. Accessed 8 August 2025
Van Eck RM, Burger TJ, Vellinga A, Schirmbeck F, De Haan L (2018) 'The relationship between clinical and personal recovery in patients with schizophrenia spectrum disorders: A systematic review and meta-analysis', Schizophrenia Bulletin 44(3):631–642. Available at: https://doi.org/10.1093/schbul/sbx088
NHS England (2019) The NHS long term plan (personalised care commitments). NHS England, London. Accessed 9 August 2025.
Entwistle VA, Watt IS (2013) A capabilities approach to person-centered care: response to open peer commentaries on 'treating patients as persons: a capabilities approach to support delivery of person-centered care'. Am J Bioeth 13(8):W1–W4. https://doi.org/10.1080/15265161.2013.812487. Accessed 27 Feb 2026
Faulkner A, Basset T (2012) A helping hand: taking peer support into the 21st century. Ment Health Soc Incl 16(1):41–47. https://doi.org/10.1108/20428301211205892. Accessed 27 Feb 2026
Fisher P (2016) Co-production: what is it and where do we begin? J Psychiatr Ment Health Nurs 23(6–7):345–346. https://doi.org/10.1111/jpm.12281. Accessed 27 Feb 2026
Franek J. (2013). Self-management support interventions for persons with chronic disease: an evidence-based analysis. Ontario health technology assessment series, 13(9), 1–60.
Freidl M, Pesola F, Konrad J, Puschner B, Kovacs AI, De Rosa C, Fiorillo A, Bording MK, Kawohl W, Rössler W, Nagy M, Munk-Jørgensen P, Slade M (2016) Effects of clinical decision topic on patients' involvement in and satisfaction with decisions and their subsequent implementation. Psychiatr Serv 67(6):658–663. https://doi.org/10.1176/appi.ps.201500083. Accessed 27 Feb 2026
Gurtner C, Schols JMGA, Lohrmann C, Hahn S (2024) 'Patients' and health professionals' perspectives regarding shared decision making in the psychiatric inpatient setting – A multiple qualitative case study', PEC Innovation, 5, Article 100352. https://doi.org/10.1016/j.pecinn.2024.100352
Health and Care Professions Council (2014) Promote and protect the interests of service users. Available at: https://www.hcpc-uk.org/students/guidance-on-conduct-and-ethics/promote-and-protect-the-interests-of-service-users/. Accessed 8 February 2025
Hummelvol JK, Karlsson B, Borg M (2015) Recovery and person-centredness in mental health services: roots of the concepts and implications for practice. Int Pract Dev J 5(Suppl):1–7. https://doi.org/10.19043/ipdj.5sp.009. Accessed 12 Feb 2025
Hurst R, Ogilvie L, Asike I, Voyce A, Carson J (2025) One ring to rule them all: Applications of the CHIME framework of mental health recovery, Social Work and Social Sciences Review, 26(1):45–64. https://doi.org/10.1921/swssr20252593
Jacobson N, Greenley D (2001) What is recovery? A conceptual model and explication. Psychiatr Serv 52(4):482–485
Joseph S (2014) Positive psychology in practice. Wiley, Hoboken
Kelly L, Ahessy B, Richardson I, moss, H. (2023) Aligning Kitwood's model of person-centred dementia care with music therapy practice. Music Ther Perspect 41:206–214
Kennedy, I. (2003) Patients are experts in their own field', BMJ 326(7402):1276–1277. Available at: https://doi.org/10.1136/bmj.326.7402.1276
Khosravi M, Azar G, Izadi R (2024) Principles and elements of patient-centredness in mental health services: a thematic analysis of a systematic review of reviews. BMJ Open Qual 13(3):1–11. https://doi.org/10.1136/bmjoq-2023-002719
Khosravi M, Azar G, Izadi R (2024) 'Principles and elements of patient-centredness in mental health services: a thematic analysis of a systematic review of reviews', BMJ Open Quality, 13(3):e002719. Available at: https://doi.org/10.1136/bmjoq-2023-002719

King's Fund (2011) Patient decision aids—an overview. The King's Fund, London. Accessed 12 May 2025

Kitwood T (1997) Dementia reconsidered: the person comes first. Open University Press, Buckingham

Kunneman M, Gionfriddo MR, Toloza FJK, Gärtner FR, Spencer-Bonilla G, Hargraves IG, Erwin PJ, Montori VM (2019) Humanistic communication in the evaluation of shared decision making: a systematic review. Patient Educ Couns 102(3):452–466. https://doi.org/10.1016/j.pec.2018.11.003

Kwame A, Petrucka P (2021) A literature-based study of patient-centered care and communication in nurse-patient interactions: barriers, facilitators, and the way forward, BMC Nursing, 20, Article 158. Available at: https://doi.org/10.1186/s12912-021-00684-2

Leamy M, Bird V, Le Boutillier C, Williams J, Slade M (2011) Conceptual framework for personal recovery in mental health: systematic review and narrative synthesis. Br J Psychiatry 199(6):445–452

Liberman RP, Kopelowicz A, Ventura J, Gutkind D (2002) Operational criteria and factors related to recovery from schizophrenia. Int Rev Psychiatry 14(4):256–272. https://doi.org/10.1080/0954026021000016905

Lombard D (2024) Three philosophies of person-centred care, from the perspectives of care workers and managers supporting older people. Social Policy & Administration. https://doi.org/10.1111/spol.13088

McCormack B, McCance T (2025) The Person-centred Nursing Framework: a mid-range theory for nursing practice. J Res Nurs 30(1):47–60. https://doi.org/10.1177/17449871241281428.

Mental Health Act 1983 (c. 20). [Online] Available at: https://www.legislation.gov.uk/ukpga/1983/20. Accessed 15 July 2026

NHS England (2016) The Five Year Forward View for Mental Health: A report from the independent Mental Health Taskforce to the NHS in England. Leeds: NHS England. Available at: https://www.england.nhs.uk/wp-content/uploads/2016/02/Mental-Health-Taskforce-FYFV-final.pdf. Accessed 8 June 2025

NICE (2026) Shared decision-making: guideline and patient decision aids. National Institute for Health and Care Excellence, London. Accessed 11 August 2025

NSUN (2020) Response to the Competence Framework for Mental Health Peer Support Workers. National Survivor User Network (NSUN), 1 November. Available at: https://www.nsun.org.uk/news/response-to-competence-framework-for-mh-psws/. Accessed: 15 July 2026

Nursing and Midwifery Council (2018) The Code: Professional standards of practice and behaviour for nurses, midwives and nursing associates. London: Nursing and Midwifery Council. Available at: https://www.nmc.org.uk/standards/code/. Accessed 19 January 2025

O'Connor AM, Stacey D, Rovner D, Holmes-Rovner M, Tetroe J, Llewellyn-Thomas H, Entwistle V, Rostom A, Fiset V, Barry M, Jones J (2001) Decision aids for people facing health treatment or screening decisions. Cochrane Database Syst Rev 3:CD001431. https://doi.org/10.1002/14651858.CD001431. Accessed 12 Feb 2025

Omundo J, Stiehl SA, Schulz M, Zingsheim A (2025) 'CHIME in practice: a qualitative exploration of CHIME framework training experiences and outcomes for service users and mental health professionals', The Journal of Mental Health Training, Education and Practice 20(3):170–183. https://doi.org/10.1108/JMHTEP-05-2024-0052

Price, B. (2020) Ethical challenges in delivering person-centred care, Primary Health Care, 30(2), pp. 34–39. Available at: doi: 10.7748/phc.2020.e1597.

Robinson S, and Isaacs A (2025) Roles, responsibilities and role challenges of lived experience workers in a regional mental health service: a qualitative study, Advances in Mental Health, 23(3), pp. 395–409. doi: 10.1080/18387357.2024.2436404.

Rogers CR (1952) Client-centered therapy. Houghton Mifflin, Boston

Sharkiya, S.H. (2023) Quality communication can improve patient-centred health outcomes among older patients: a rapid review, BMC Health Services Research, 23, Article 886. Available at: doi: 10.1186/s12913-023-09869-8.

Slade M (2009) Personal recovery and mental illness: a guide for mental health professionals. Cambridge University Press, Cambridge

Slade M (2017) Implementing shared decision-making in routine mental health care. World Psychiatry 16(2):146–153

Stanyon M, Ryank K, Dilks J, Hartshorn K, Ingley P, Kumar B, Mahalinggappa S, Mullins E, Misquitta O, Sidwell A, Dave S (2024) Impact of involvement in mental health professional education on patient educators: a qualitative systematic review. BMJ Open 14:e084314. https://doi.org/10.1136/bmjopen-2024-084314. Accessed 12 Feb 2025

Stuart SR, Tansey L, Quayle E (2017) What we talk about when we talk about recovery: a systematic review. J Ment Health 26(4):291–304

Terry J, Garner J (2024) Meaningful service user involvement. In: Wright KM, McKeown M (eds) Essentials of mental health nursing, 2nd edn. SAGE, London

The Health Foundation (2016) Person-centred care made simple: What everyone should know about person-centred care. London: The Health Foundation. Available at: https://www.health.org.uk/resources-and-toolkits/quick-guides/person-centred-care-made-simple

White S, Foster R, Marks J, Morshead R, Goldsmith L, Barlow S, Sin J, Gillard S, Lloyd-Evans B (2020) The effectiveness of one-to-one peer support in mental health services: a systematic review and meta-analysis'. BMC Psychiatry 20(1):534. https://doi.org/10.1186/s12888-020-02923-3. Accessed 12 Feb 2025

Yao, L. and Kabir, R. (2023) Person-Centered Therapy (Rogerian Therapy). In: StatPearls [Internet]. Treasure Island, FL: StatPearls Publishing. Available at: https://www.ncbi.nlm.nih.gov/books/NBK589708/

Yu Y, Shen M, Niu L, Liu Y, Xiao S, Tebes JK (2022) The relationship between clinical recovery and personal recovery among people living with schizophrenia: a serial mediation model and the role of disability and quality of life. Schizophr Res 239:168–175. https://doi.org/10.1016/j.schres.2021.11.043. Accessed 12 Feb 2025

Models of Communication

Case Study

Muhammed presented to the Accident and Emergency Department with his daughter- and son-in-law. They discussed their concern regarding his growing anxiety over the last 5 months.

Muhammed described himself as being increasingly worried about his finances and business. He describes poor sleep, lack of concentration and a lack of focus when doing tasks within his business. Muhammed was involved in a disagreement with a customer in his shop recently, who he had known for a long period of time. His daughter- and son-in-law state that he was very uncharacteristic in the way that he spoke to this customer, as they had known each other for a long period of time. When you ask for more details about what was said, his daughter says he was very 'cold' and 'rude' to the customer. Muhammed becomes very tearful at this comment.

Muhammed reports that he has been drinking more caffeine than usual. Muhammed reports that he is struggling to keep active and engaged, and caffeine is helping him with this. During the initial assessment, Muhammed spent much of the time staring at the floor with very fleeting eye contact. He sat slouched back in the chair in the corner of the room, facing out towards the window and away from his family. He did not initiate conversation, and his answers were short and to the point.

What are your initial concerns about Muhammed?
How would you start building a relationship with Muhammed?

R. Bage, *Mental Health Skills for Adult Nurses & Non-Specialist Healthcare Workers*, https://doi.org/10.1007/978-3-032-32835-9_3

Foundations of Therapeutic Communication

Therapeutic relationships are often seen as the fundamental basis of a mental health nursing identity (O'Brien 2001). Literature about therapeutic relationships was more commonly seen in the 1950's onwards, work around therapeutic relationships can indeed be seen since the asylum era (O'Brien 2001).

Allderidge (1985) provides two case studies that start to look at therapeutic relationships. James Norris was admitted in 1800 and was described as '...the most violent and dangerous patient that Bethlem had every encountered'. He was restrained by a custom-made iron cafe for almost 10 years, which maybe demonstrates everything that many of us find difficult about the period of Asylums. Allderidge (1985) describes two aspects of Norris' treatment at the time. During his confinement, Norris read books and newspapers and played with his cat. These start to demonstrate there were humane and caring practices, aimed at meeting some of James's basic human needs (O'Brien 2001; Allderidge 1985).

Allderidge (1985) also discusses the case of James Tilly Matthews who was admitted earlier than Norris in 1797. He appears to have been less violent than Norris but was convinced he was emperor of the world (and detained due to concerns that he was a risk to the Royal Family). James was a talented artist and would often stay up at night drawing. In 1810, he submitted a competition entry for designing the new Bethlem Hospital and was paid for his work (O'Brien 2001). Some of his work can be seen in the book 'The Discovery of the Art of the Insane' (Macgregor 1989). Overall, there was evidence that his interest, and skill, in art was encouraged whilst at the Bethlem.

Slightly later, Florence Nightingale, in the late 1800s, discussed the importance of 'always sitting in the patient's view...continuously raise his eyes to see you' and 'never speak to an invalid from behind...nor when he is doing anything' (Karimi and Masoudi Alavi 2015).

The more modern ideas of therapeutic care were from nursing theorists in the United States (O'Brien 2001). Sullivan and Reusch were key figures in interpersonal theory and communication and discussed the importance of communication in therapeutic benefit (Sharma and Gupta 2023). Peplau's work in the 'A conceptual Frame of Reference for Psychodynamic Nursing' has frequently been linked as the earliest link between nursing and therapeutic relationships (Peplau 1952, 1988). It is important to note that Peplau's work was for all nurses, and not just mental health nurses (O'Brien 2001). Her work refers to the therapeutic value of nursing, describing it as '...a significant, therapeutic, interpersonal process' (O'Brien 2001).

Case Study

There are some significant signs going on for Mohammed. He describes poor sleep, lack of concentration, lack of focus and a recent disagreement with a customer. These all appear to be unusual symptoms for him. His family also give more detail that his behaviour has been very uncharacteristic. There are also concerns about caffeine, eye contact and his body language within the clinic room. You may notice that he is not initiating speech, and his answers are short.

It can be challenging to develop a relationship with somebody who has poor eye contact, closed body language and limited speech. However, you may want to focus on building a connection with Mohammed. Sometimes it can be useful to identify a shared interest to try and engage him in further conversation. You may want to make sure that you are not filling Muhammed's silence, as this can often be easy to do. It may also be beneficial to try and build a relationship over a 'task'—this might be a game, crossword or something simple like choosing a sandwich. We will all tackle this in different ways, but it is important to reflect how you may want to do it.

Peplau identified the concept of the 'nurse–patient' relationship in her 1952 book 'Interpersonal Relations in Nursing'. Peplau also went on to develop a model for nurses based on the therapeutic interpersonal process—you may have seen this referred to as 'Peplau's theory of interpersonal relations model'. This model is made up of four phases:

Orientation.
Identification.
Exploitation.
Resolution (Peplau 1988).

In modern health care, we can consider that therapeutic relationship is the relationship between a professional and service user. It is the relationship by which the professional hopes to engage and effect change in a service user. You may also see it referred to as the helping alliance, therapeutic alliance and the working alliance.

BOND Framework

Baughan and Smith (2013) developed a framework based on the analysis of stories from nursing students, registered practitioners and service users. The framework has eighteen caring indicators which are grouped into four 'bonded' themes (Baughan and Smith 2013). The framework gets the label 'BOND' after the four grouped themes:

B = being and becoming.
O = overcoming obstacles.
N = noticing.
D = doing.

Being and Becoming

This is an important theme for compassionate care. Baughan and Smith (2013) state the importance of nurses to be adaptable, creative and ready to learn. They also discuss the need for nurses to be a caring empathetic presence for those who they work with, which is an additional requirement for nurses (and other health-care professionals). Being and becoming looks at the importance of emotional intelligence in nursing practitioners (Barker and Emile 2024; Baughan and Smith 2013).

Overcoming Obstacles

It is important that as clinicians, we feel able to overcome the obstacles that might impact our compassionate care. In mental health care, or any kind of health care, this might be factors such as stress, workload or organisational constraints.

Noticing

Noticing involves the person-centred care that we see as important in mental health practice. This might be about actively listening to your service user and making sure that you are picking up all the important elements of the conversations.

Doing

This might involve elements such as practical support, communication or advocacy with the service user. These are the practical steps that you might take.

Task

What elements of the 'BOND' framework could you take on board for your own practice?

Building Rapport

Rapport could be considered the harmonious relationship that you have with a service user, and something you can build on for collaboration (Butt 2021). However, whilst rapport is essential to the service user–provider relationship, it is often poorly defined (English et al. 2022).

Many of us will have our own way of building rapport with a service user. My own approach is often to use humour or laughter to try and build that bridge. Work by Butt (2021) suggests using discussion about occupation and social history at the start of a conversation (Butt 2021). Importantly, simple and kind gestures are crucial to build rapport with service users, such as a cup of tea or other act of kindness (English et al. 2022).

Models and Approaches

There are multiple communication models which are used in practice, some of which will be covered below.

Communication Models

Calgary-Cambridge Model

The Calgary-Cambridge Model (Silverman et al. 2013) identifies five stages for the consultation which are listed below:

- Initiate the session.
- Gather history.
- Physical exam.
- Explain and plan.
- Close the session.

It also identifies two themes that should be running throughout the consultation:

1. Good communication and building rapport.
2. Overt structure and good flow throughout (Silverman et al. 2013).

Verbal micro skills are also important within mental health services. This looks at things wider than just what is said, but also the tone of voice, volume of voice and the speed of what you are saying (Barker and Emile 2024). Paralinguistics looked at the importance of verbalising comments such as 'ahh' uh huh' and 'ermm'. These can be useful for demonstrating your concentration and engagement in the conversation and continuing to encourage the service user to talk. Similarly, tools such as focussing, reflecting and probing may also help demonstrate your engagement with service users and encourage further discussion (Barker and Emile 2024).

Trauma-Informed Practice

Trauma involved care is a system approach that understands and responds to the prevalence and impact of trauma and adversity. This happens in a way to cause no further harm.

Trauma can be defined as:

> Individual trauma results from an event, series of events, or set of circumstances that is experienced by an individual as physically or emotionally harmful or life threatening and that has lasting adverse effects on the individual's functioning and mental, physical, social, emotional, or spiritual well-being. (US Substance Abuse and Mental Health Service Administration)

Almost 1/3 of young people in the UK experience trauma during childhood or adolescence and this doubles their risk of developing a range of different mental health conditions (Torjesen 2019). Equally, around 1 in 3 adults in England have reported they have experienced at least one traumatic event. This could include road accidents, natural disasters, serious illness or abuse (Mental Health Foundation 2022).

The 4 Rs of trauma-informed care are included in Table 1 (NHS England 2025):

For example, in ward-based care this would look like focussing on relationships which service users can trust and feel safe. You would focus on providing a warm and welcoming environment, where you feel confident in providing a trauma-informed, compassionate response (NHS England 2025). Further to this, the Office for Health Improvement & Disparities has produced six principles of trauma information practice, which is included in Table 2.

It is important to consider what trauma-informed care is not. This should not just look like a repackage of existing services, as true trauma-informed care requires a significant cultural change from leadership and the opportunity for reflection and supervision. Equally, we should not simply assume that all people within mental health services have experienced trauma. People may not have experienced trauma, or they may be unwilling to disclose or discuss any prior experiences of trauma (NHS England 2025). We should not forget that people will develop mental ill health for a number of different reasons, and this does not have to be trauma related.

What might trauma-informed care look like for you?

You might ensure that you talk to a service user about why you are asking sensitive questions.

Table 1 Trauma-informed care

Realise	All people have a basic understanding of trauma and how it can impact individuals, families and communities
Recognise	Professionals within services can recognise trauma, and how it can impact individuals and families
Respond	Organisation can respond by implementing and practising a trauma-informed approach
Resist retraumatisation	Organisational practices can compound trauma. Organisations will work to ensure that this does not happen within their organisation.

Table 2 Trauma-information practice

Safety	It is important that people feel safe, and it is important that clinicians are asking what is needed for service users to feel safe. It is important to try and attempt any further retraumatisation for the students
Trustworthiness	Transparent within organisation's policies and procedures. Staff and organisation are explaining what they are doing and why. Expectations are being made clear.
Choice	Ensuring service users are supported in shared decision-making, choice and goal setting. Listening to the needs and wishes of service users and staff. Explaining choices clearly and transparently.
Collaboration	Using formal and information peer support Organisations asking service user and staff what they need and identifying how these things can be met collaboratively Focussing on working alongside service users and involving service users on the delivery of services
Empowerment	Ensure that service users have a strong voice in decision-making Making sure that feelings and concerns of staff and service users are validated Ensuring practitioners are listened to, and their wants and needs are listened to People are supported to make decisions and take action People who have experienced trauma may feel powerless and isolated by previous experiences.
Cultural consideration	Offering gender responsive services Considering the healing value of traditional cultural connections Incorporating policies, protocols and processes that are responsive to the needs of the service users

Adapted from Office for Health Improvement and Disparities (2022)

You might enquire further when a person refuses their cervical smear test. You might see if you can put any adjustments in place to help them attend.

If somebody books an appointment, but cancels, you might ask with compassion whether there is anything further you could do to help them attend their appointment.

You might see somebody struggling in Accident and Emergency. You might ask them if there is anything that has worked previously when they have attended A + E. You might enquire if there is a room for them to sit if they are distressed.

Case Study

You are a practice nurse meeting Emma, who has come in her for routine cervical screening. She has not attended two of these appointments, so you are pleased she has attended.

When you call Emma, she seems startled and gives no eye contact. She walks very slowly and spends the walk to the room staring at the floor. You introduce yourself, but she sits looking out of the window clutching her bag and coat.

Emma offers short answers to your questions, staring either out the window or at the floor. When you ask her to undress from the waist down, you notice her getting tearful and her breathing becomes faster. Emma states that 'she can't do this' and 'she's sorry'. She goes to grab her coat and says, 'she has had bad experiences' and she stands up.

You try and acknowledge her concerns—'Oh Emma, thanks for telling me. I am so sorry you find this uncomfortable. Lots and lots of people find this uncomfortable, and we can do this at your pace'.

You invite Emma to sit back down, and you then proceed to go through the appointment. You try and make sure you offer her choice about inserting the speculum herself or having someone else present. You offer to move the appointment so she can have some time to prepare.

Emma chooses to go ahead with the appointment, but she asks you if she can put some music on to reorientate herself. She also asks that you talk to her throughout the procedure, so nothing is a surprise. You ask her to undress on her bottom half and she bursts into tears. You immediately stop and sit down with her. You again validate her reaction and remind her that it is her choice to go ahead. You tell her again that lots of people find this difficult.

She asks if she can have someone in the room too, that she can look at and talk to. You find one of the students and she comes to support. With reassurance, and the student nurse talking throughout, Emma is able to complete the procedure. She thanks you and says she is proud of herself. You remind her that there are support services which might help her and make sure you document the extra support she needs for next appointment.

Reflective Questions

What signs indicated that Emma did not feel safe?
What strategies were used within the case study to make Emma feel safe?
What other strategies may be available to healthcare practitioners?
How did the nurse communicate with Emma?
What other strategies could you take to support Emma?
How could you take steps to avoid retraumatisation?
What support might the nurse need if she needs to support trauma-informed care sustainably?

Discussion

In Emma's situation, you would want to ensure that you follow the basic principles of trauma-informed care. You do not need to know any further information on what has happened, you just need to act on the behaviours you are seeing (tearfulness, lack of eye contact, reluctant engagement, cancelling of appointments).

The nurse in this case study did a good job of making sure she was listened to and built trust even in a very short consultation. She listened very attentively Emma, which was useful in understanding her reluctance and she validated the thoughts and feelings of Emma.

However, it is easy to see how this trauma-informed care might get missed. Practice nursing is a very busy, time pressured role and there is a pressure to stay on track with appointments. It really requires a change of perspective.

De-escalation

Common causes of conflict can include:

- Long waiting times.
- Perceived long waiting times.
- Unreasonable demands and expectations.
- Heightened sense of vulnerability or anxiety.
- Alcohol/drug intake.
- Other patient factors (e.g. post-traumatic experiences).
- Ward environments.
- Staff–patient interactions (Lavelle et al. 2024; NHS Tayside n.d.).

De-escalation could be defined as:

> A collective term for a range of interwoven staff-delivered components comprising communication, self-regulation, assessment, actions and safety maintenance, which aims to extinguish or reduce patient aggression/agitation irrespective of its cause and improve staff-patient relationships whilst eliminating or minimising coercion or restriction. (Hallett and Dickens 2017)

Verbal de-escalation does not happen alone. De-escalation is an important combination of verbal, gestural and non-verbal communication (Lavelle et al. 2024). However, you may find that verbal communication is often highlighted as the most important factor in de-escalation (Lavelle et al. 2024).

Safewards Model

The Safewards Model is shown in Fig. 1 and can be accessed in from the safewards.net website (Safewards 2026).

Further detail on how you can use the Safewards model (Safewards 2026) is shown in Table 3.

Another option is the 'Talk Down' approach, which goes alongside the Safewards intervention. The 'Talk Down' approach is a three-step process, which draws on previously developed techniques and details.

Delimiting—establishing safety and getting started.
Clarifying—eliciting and hearing the patient, establishing the nature of the problem.

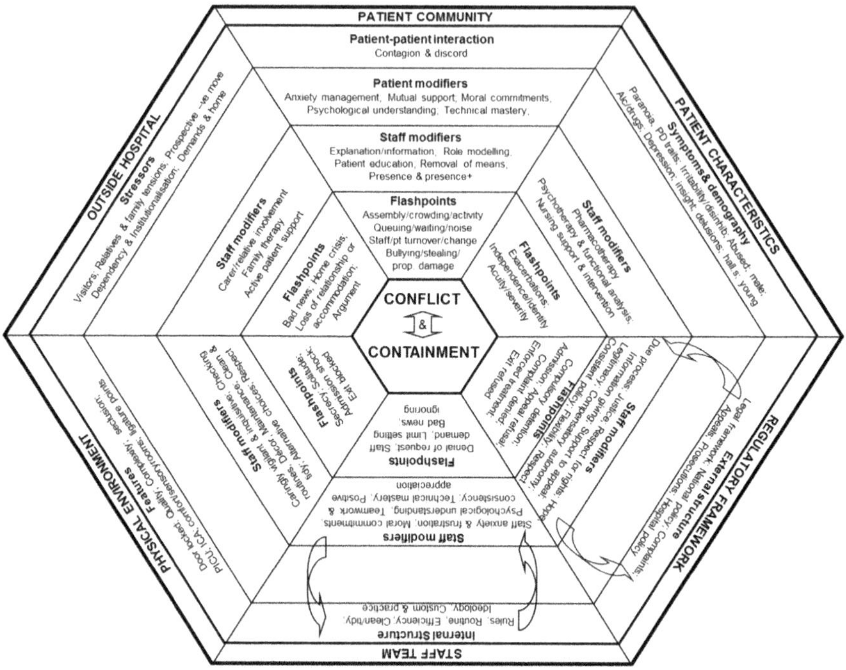

Fig. 1 The Safewards Model

Resolving—addressing the issue via appeal negotiation, compromise or providing choices.

Another option, from Lavelle et al. (2024) gives options to look at de-escalation from a trauma-informed lens (Table 4).

Working with Specific Presentations

Dementia

Brooker and Latham (2015) conceptualised person-centred care, see Table 5, for dementia in the form of a formulation, using the acronym 'VIPS', and discussed earlier in this book.

$$PCC(\text{person} - \text{centred care}) = \text{V} + \text{I} + \text{P} + \text{S}$$

Brooker and Latham (2015) also discuss the importance as seeing the world from the perspective of the person with dementia, rather than just the carer (as these perspectives can vary). Practitioners should not forget a person is viewing the world through the added filter of their cognitive difficulties. Brooker and Latham (2015) highlighted the following two concepts:

Table 3 Safewards Model

Originating domains	Flashpoints—examples	Staff modifiers—examples
Staff team or internal team structures This looks at how staff can manage their own feels, and the consistently in the setting	When staff set limits to service user behaviour	Ensure compassionate and careful communication when staff are asking service users to do (or stop) doing something
Physical environment domain The nicer the ward is in terms of equipment, furniture and decor, the more comfortable service users will feel. This also includes the line of sight you have to service users on your ward	Service users being isolate for significant periods of time Furniture or equipment being broken Environments that are poorly decorated or depressing The first few days of an admission (to any setting) when there is a culture shock	Ensuring that priority is given to the decor and repair needs of your work setting Staff knowing where service users are an ensuring option to make choices
Outside hospital domain Consideration of outside forces for service users such as money worries, drug and alcohol use	Arguing with service users and friends Service users coping with significant life events such as bereavement or illness Service users receiving bad news Crisis at home, away from the ward environment	Staff being aware of a service user's friends and family Staff supporting friends and families Ensuring you are aware of stressors that are impacting your patient group off the ward.
Patient characteristics There are three characteristics that are more likely to cause conflict—paranoia or hallucinations, those who have difficulty relating to others, demographic factors	Staff to reorientate and guide others Staff giving restrictions or barriers Perceived loss of liberties, e.g. access to smoking or vaping	Responsive treatments given Staff given good explanations on treatment plans and guidance Compassionate communication
Regulatory framework Ensuring all professional and legal policies and frameworks are followed e.g. Mental Health Act and Mental Capacity Act	When the realities of becoming confined against your will are realised, e.g. mental health act or mental capacity act When service users feel that staff are abusing their power	Ensuring rights are followed Ensuring service users are given all the information they need including how to appeal

Person-centred attitudes: carers to embrace the ideas of person-centred and relationship-centred care. Clinicians must want to put these principles in practice (Pulsford and Smith et al. 2024).

Compassionate approach: this looks at the professional's personal manner with their skills at delivering individualised care. The professionals must be reassuring,

Table 4 De-escalation from a trauma-informed lens

Acute phase	
Respect personal space	To allow for good dialogue, clinicians should not violate the patient's personal space Personal space can be established by clinician's keeping good distance and allowing plenty of time
Create focus	Clinicians to give focussed attention—the clinicians must not be engaging with anyone other than the patient
Change context	Either creating a diversion for the patient, or by giving new meaning to the situation This can be a good turning point for the patient

Relationship phase	
Show empathy	Empathy is an important element for successful de-escalation Clinician to put themselves in the patient's shows Supporting autonomy
Understand the patient	Once dialogue has begun, make a determined effort to understand the patient's point of view or perspective Keep listening to the patient story and experiences Clinicians need to stay open and curious
Align expectations	Find a common solution to a problem by first aligning expectations. Shared decision-making
Evaluate the process	Encourage atmosphere where staff and service users can reflect on what has happened and learn from the situation Do not interpret the behaviour of others

Table 5 VIPS

V	Valuing people with dementia and those who care for them
I	Treating people as individuals
P	Looking at the world from the perspective of the person with dementia
S	A positive social environment in which the person living with dementia can experience relative wellbeing

open and reaching out of the person. Professionals need to act with creativity (Pulsford and Smith et al. 2024).

Personality Disorders

An interesting article from Dr. Entwistle summarising research discusses the differences in language use. Research suggests that those with darker personality traits may use more hostile or negative language—including more swear words and anger words. People with darker personality traits also use fewer socially connected works such as 'we'. People in distress will use more self-focussed language and more negative emotion words. This is as our language tracks our attention, emotion and thought (Entwistle 2025).

A study completed by Mangalik et al. (2024) studied social media posts from people with personality disorder compared to those from the general population. From this, they examined how people explore their self-beliefs. From this, they found that those in the personality disorder group shared self-beliefs more frequently on online forums. Within this, their wording was often more negative and extreme such as 'mental health', "symptoms' and 'medication'. Alongside this, they also used more emotional descriptors such as 'suicidal', "abusive' and 'hurt'.

Ensuring you use open communication and working with the trauma-informed care guidance when working with people who have a personality disorder is key. A 2015 study found that open communication was important to ensure a therapeutic relationship is maintained (Sulzer et al. 2016). People who have a personality disorder have often experience poor relationships and inconsistent relationships in the past, and so making sure you are transparent about the length of your involvement is a clear step that shows you are open and can be trusted.

Non-verbal, Cultural and Accessibility Considerations

Non-verbal Communication

Non-verbal communication skills are often broken down into haptics, proxemics and kinesics (Barker and Emile 2024).

Haptics

Haptics refers to the way that people respond through touch of feel. It can also relate to the idea of proprioception (Barker and Emile 2024).

Proxemics

Proxemics focussing in about the position, distance and space (Barker and Emile 2024).

Kinesics

Kinesics focusses on communication through gestures. This can include elements such as facial expressions, gestures, eye movement and posture (Barker and Emile 2024).

There is culturally specific meaning in our non-verbal behaviours (Lorié et al. 2017). The ability to understand our non-verbal communication is important for our cross-cultural communication (Pang et al. 2024).

Ekman and Friesen (1978) identified six universal facial expressions of emotion. These are generally well understood across cultures and are listed in Table 6.

At times, we do use our non-verbal communication within our diagnostic criteria (the ICD-11). Please see some examples below:

Schizophrenia—catatonic posturing; agitation; posturing.

Table 6 Facial expressions of emotion

Emotion	Signs
Happiness	Corners of the lips draw upward and nasolabial folds become prominent Lower eyelid raises and wrinkles appear around the eyes
Sadness	Lips tremble or corners draw downward Tears may appear in eyes Inner brows are raised and often drawn together
Surprise	Jaw drops Opening the mouth without tension eyes open widely Brows are raised, high and curved Forehead wrinkles horizontally throughout
Anger	Lips tightly closed Eyelids tense Brows are lowered and drawn close together Wrinkling appears vertically between the brows
Disgust	Upper lip raises and nose wrinkles Lower eyelid moves upward Brows are lowered
Fear	Lips tense, stretch and draw back Eyes open with lower lid tense and upper lid raised Brows are raised Drawn close together; forehead wrinkles horizontally in the Centre only

When we look at the non-verbal communication, we need to consider whether it matches the verbal communication of the service user. Their verbal communication may be congruent or incongruent to the verbal communication. For example, if a patient presented in Accident and Emergency.

Non-verbal communication is an important tool in your overall assessment of a service user. If your service user presented stating they had no history of self-harm, but you can physically see marks on the arm indicative of this, then we may consider them at a greater risk.

Egan (1977) offers maybe one of the most written about model of communication. This is a strategy to position in the body most helpfully in therapeutic interactions. SOLER, Egan's model, stands for: sit squarely, open posture, lean forward, eye contact and relax. A more contemporary acronym was provided by Stickley (2011) and there is value in considering how your communication fits in the SURETY framework

Sit at an angle.
Uncross arms and legs.
Relax.
Eye contact.
Touch.
Your intuition.

Non-verbal Communication of Staff

Research, looking into relationships with Psychiatrists, has suggested that rapport with your service users is impacted by three different non-verbal elements—attentiveness, positivity–negativity and coordination (Tickle-Degnan and Gavett). This gives us three clear elements to focus on when first engaging with a service user.

Attentiveness

This looks at the capability of the practitioner to focus on the interaction between professional and service user. Service users will pick up if the professional looks distracted or disinterested in the exchange, and this will undermine the rapport developed. Focussing on non-verbal communication strategies such as eye contact and nodding will support in ensuring the service user is aware that you are solely focussing on them (Tickle and Degnan).

Positivity–Negativity

This looks at the specifics within the interactions between professional and service user. Service users will look out for signs that professionals are enjoying the company—such as laughing, leaning forward on the chair and having an open posture. Service users will focus on negative signs such as closed posture, physical distance or barriers which may be described as hostility (Tickle and Degnan).

Coordination

Coordination looks at the non-verbal behaviour similarity between professional and service user. You may want to think of this as the mirroring of behaviours. Service users will look at elements such as the return of a smile, eye contact at the same moment or positional moves which mirror each other (Tickle and Degnen).

Boundaries, Confidentiality and Trust

The Mental Health Nurse Handbook (NHS England 2022) identifies a 14-item list of mental health nursing requirements that are not about finances or budgets. Lots of these focus on boundaries, relationships and communication. These provide a good framework to work with when working with service users presenting with mental health difficulties:

1. Listen to the service user.
2. Show kindness and compassion.
3. Take your time to make a judgement—gather all the facts.
4. Collaborative information.
5. Work in partnership with service users, your MDT and wider system partners such as local authority, education and social care.
6. Do the very best you can—what you would do for your own family.
7. Be honest about what you cannot do.
8. Be hopeful.
9. Show people they matter.
10. Notice the small things, notice all things.
11. See the person, not just the mental health diagnosis.
12. Be determined.
13. Be visible.
14. Seek feedback.

Boundaries

Reflective Questions
What are your boundaries in your work?
Do they ever change? If they do, why is this?

All health professionals, including mental health nurses, have boundaries in their professional workspace. This is a healthy approach to support safe interactions between service user, their carers and staff members. Boundaries can often be unclear, however. In a modern workplace, there are boundaries between personal, cultural, professional and virtual settings which might not always be clear (Hungerford 2025). How many times have you checked your virtual collaboration and communication platform, like MS Teams, out of hours?

Relational boundaries are an important factor of healthcare practice, with there often being a sizeable power differential between professional and service user (Birger and Nadan 2022). The service users we see may be in a vulnerable or compromising situation, and the nurse or health professional is there in a position of knowledge (Hungerford 2025). Relational boundaries act as the rules of engagement that cover the way we interact. This can include factors such as physical, psychological, social and sexual, and the impact of this appropriateness on speech, behaviour or activity (Thomson et al. 2024).

Professional boundaries have been described as unclear in mental health services (Thomson et al. 2024). In mental health, professionals can both support their service users, but also often have the power to detain them. In this scenario, it is useful to relate back to work of Dowding (1996). Dowding (1996) discussed the concepts of 'power to' and 'power over'. In mental health, power over might be around using social incentives to bring around change—a carrot and stick approach. Power to looks more about the ability the power of an outcome, such as a service user telling a staff member about their suicidal thoughts.

Confidentiality

Confidentiality is an important part of mental health care (Conlon et al. 2020); however, it can often be seen as a barrier to working with families and carers (Doody et al. 2017). Family involvement during mental illness is still poorly implemented, despite evidence highlighting its importance (Hansson et al. 2022). On many occasions, clinicians lack confidence in knowing when to share information and when not to. Carers and families play a crucial role in recovery, and we should involve them as much as the service user consents to within our practice.

Lindon (2007) highlighted some of the issues faced by carers who are trying to support those with a mental health illness:

- The unpredictability of caring for someone with a mental health problem.
- The stigma of mental illness.
- Confidentiality and information-sharing conflicts with mental health professional.
- The constant fear of a loved one's suicide.
- The lack of specialised respite or 'sitting services.

Key Learning Points

Therapeutic relationships are the foundations of the communication and for the care that we give. We should never forget the very important aspects of our soft skills such as introductions, active listening, empathy and validation.

We should all work to becoming more trauma-informed in our practice. I am confident that not many of us go into work to increase or revisit somebody's trauma. We should all do everything we can to avoid retraumatisation.

We should all be paying close attention to non-verbal and verbal communication. Non-verbal communication is key within any conversations, and we should ensure we work to feel confident in aspects of non-verbal communication that we may see in practice.

We should ensure that we feel confident in skills to keep a key professional boundary and being transparent about this relation to our service users.

It is important to remember that de-escalation is a skill, and not something that comes naturally. We will all have different approaches to de-escalate situations, but there are other models and tools that can help us develop that skill.

We need to all be careful in our own communication. Please think about how your communication may come across and how that may be received by service users and their families. I say this as someone who has, as told by a mentor on my first placement as a student, a 'naturally disinterested' face.

Conclusion

This chapter has shown the role of communication across mental health and importance of using communication to build relationships based on trust and safety.

Central to this chapter has been that non-verbal communication has as much importance as verbal communication. Non-verbal communication skills, and our knowledge of how we come across, can be important in ensuring that service users feel respectful and safe.

Equally, this chapter has highlighted the importance of skilled communication in moments of challenging behaviour, high emotion or conflict.

Theme of this chapter reinforces that communication is key in communicating with service users who are presenting will mental ill health. This is regardless of profession, location or service. By understanding the key frameworks in communication and balancing with soft skill and interpersonal skills, practitioners have the opportunity to confidently develop therapeutic relationships that allow service users to feel safe and supported.

References

Allderidge P (1985) Bedlam: fact of fantasy? In: Bynum WF, Porter R, Sherpard M (eds) The anatomy of madness: essays in the history of psychiatry, vol II. Institutions and Society, Tavistock, London, pp 17–33

Barker S, Emile G (2024) Compassionate communication in mental health care. In: Wright KM, McKeown M (eds) Essentials of mental health nursing, 2nd edn. Sage Publications, London, pp 403–421

Baughan J, Smith A (2013) Compassion, caring and communication: skills for nursing practice. Taylor and Francis, Hoboken

Birger L, Nadan Y (2022) Social workers and refugee service users (re)constructing their relationships in a hostile political climate. J Soc Work 22(2):402–421. https://doi.org/10.1177/14680173211009739. Accessed 7 Feb 2026

Brooker D Latham I (2015) Person-Centred Dementia Care: Making Services Better with the VIPS Framework. 2nd edn. London: Jessica Kingsley Publishers.

Butt MF (2021) Approaches to building rapport with patients. Clin Med 21(6):e662–e663. https://doi.org/10.7861/clinmed.2021-0264. Accessed 7 Feb 2026

Conlon D, Raeburn T, Wand T (2020) Decision-making processes of a nurse working in mental health, regarding disclosure of confidential personal health information of a patient assessed as posing a risk. Collegian 28(3). https://doi.org/10.1016/j.colegn.2020.08.010. Accessed 7 Feb 2026

Doody O, Butler MP, Lions R, Newman D (2017) Families' experiences of involvement in care planning in mental health services: an integrative literature review. J Psychiatr Ment Health Nurs 24(6):412–430. https://doi.org/10.1111/jpm.12369. Accessed 7 Feb 2026

Dowding K (1996) Power. University of Minnesota Press, Minneapolis

Egan G (1977) The skilled helper. Brooks/Cole, Monterey

Ekman P, Friesen WV (1978) Facial action coding system (FACS) [Database record]. APA PsycTests

English W, Gott M, Robinson J (2022) The meaning of rapport for patients, families, and healthcare professionals: A scoping review, Patient Educ Couns, 105(1):2–14. https://doi.org/10.1016/j.pec.2021.06.003.

Entwistle C (2025) People with personality disorders often use language differently – our research reveals how', The Conversation. Available at: https://theconversation.com/people-with-personality-disorders-often-use-language-differently-our-research-reveals-how Accessed 19 February 2026

Hallett N, Dickens GL (2017) De-escalation of aggressive behaviour in healthcare settings: concept analysis. Int J Nurs Stud 75:10–20. https://doi.org/10.1016/j.ijnurstu.2017.07.003. Accessed 7 Feb 2026

Hansson KM, Romøren M, Weimand B, Heiervang KS, Hestmark L, Landeweer EGM, Pedersen R (2022) The duty of confidentiality during family involvement: ethical challenges and possible solutions in the treatment of persons with psychotic disorders. BMC Psychiatry 22(1). https://doi.org/10.1186/s12888-022-04461-6. Accessed 7 Feb 2026

Hungerford CL (2025) Boundaries in health settings: a discursive paper. Issues Ment Health Nurs 46(10):1–8. https://doi.org/10.1080/01612840.2025.2551686

Karimi H, Masoudi Alavi N (2015) Florence nightingale's nursing theory as literature review. Nurs Midwifery Stud 4(2):e29475. Accessed 7 Feb 2026

Lavelle M, Ferreira AL, Dixen S, Berring LL (2024) De-escalation in mental health care settings. In: Hallett N, Whittington R, Richter D, Eneje E (eds) Coercion and violence in mental health settings. Springer, Cham. https://doi.org/10.1007/978-3-031-61224-4_15. Accessed 7 Feb 2026

Lindon D (2007) 5 key facts about mental health carers. Available from: https://professionals.carers.org/sites/default/files/media/5-key-facts-on-mh-carers-final-2825. Accessed 7 Feb 2026

Lorié Á, Reinero DA, Phillips M, Zhang L, Riess H (2017) Culture and nonverbal expressions of empathy in clinical settings: a systematic review. Patient Educ Couns 100(3):411–424. https://doi.org/10.1016/j.pec.2016.09.018. Accessed 7 Feb 2026

MacGregor JM (1989) The Discovery of the Art of the Insane. Princeton, NJ: Princeton University Press.

Mangalik S, Eichstaedt JC, Giorgi S, Mun J, Ahmed F, Gill G, Ganesan AV, Subrahmanya S, Soni N, Clouston SAP, Schwartz HA (2024) 'Robust language-based mental health assessments in time and space through social media', npj Digital Medicine, 7, Article 109. Available at: https://doi.org/10.1038/s41746-024-01100-0.

Mental Health Foundation (2022) The impact of traumatic events on mental health. Available at: https://www.mentalhealth.org.uk/explore-mental-health/publications/impact-traumatic-events-mental-health Accessed 18 March 2025

NHS England (2022) The mental health nurse's handbook. Available at: https://www.england.nhs.uk/long-read/the-mental-health-nurses-handbook/ Accessed 7 February 2025

NHS England (2025) Trauma-informed, harm-aware inpatient care. Available at: https://www.england.nhs.uk/long-read/trauma-informed-harm-aware-inpatient-care/. Accessed 7 Feb 2026

NHS Tayside (n.d.) Defusing potential conflict & aggression (Toolbox Talk No. HS-004, Version 1.1). NHS Tayside. Available at: NHS Tayside internal publication/PDF. Accessed 7 May 2026

O'Brien AJ (2001) The therapeutic relationship: historical development and contemporary significance. J Psychiatr Ment Health Nurs 8(2):129–137. https://doi.org/10.1046/j.1365-2850.2001.00367. Accessed 7 Feb 2026

Office for Health Improvement & Disparities (2022) Working definition and principles of trauma-informed practice. Available at: https://www.gov.uk/government/publications/working-definition-of-trauma-informed-practice/working-definition-of-trauma-informed-practice. Accessed 7 Feb 2026

Pang HT, Zhou X, Chu M (2024) Cross-cultural differences in using nonverbal behaviors to identify indirect replies. J Nonverbal Behav 48(2):323–344

Peplau HE (1952/1988) Interpersonal relations in nursing/A conceptual frame of reference for psychodynamic nursing. Putnam, New York. Reprint 1988

Safewards (2026) Safewards Model (website). Available at: https://www.safewards.net. Accessed 7 Feb 2026

Sharma NP, Gupta V (2023) Therapeutic Communication. In: StatPearls [Internet]. Treasure Island (FL): StatPearls Publishing. Available at: https://www.ncbi.nlm.nih.gov/books/NBK567775/

Silverman J, Kurtz S, Draper J (2013) Skills for communicating with patients (Calgary–Cambridge guide), 3rd edn. Radcliffe, Abingdon

Stickley T (2011) From SOLER to SURETY…. Nurse Educ Pract 11(6):395–398

Substance Abuse and Mental Health Services Administration (2024) Trauma and violence. [Online] Samhsa.gov. Available at: https://www.samhsa.gov/mental-health/trauma-violence. Accessed 7 Feb 2026

Sulzer SH, Muenchow E, Potvin A, Harris J, Gigot G (2016) Improving patient-centered communication of the borderline personality disorder diagnosis. J Ment Health 25(1):5–9. https://doi.org/10.3109/09638237.2015.1022253. Accessed 7 Feb 2026

Thomson AE, Karpa J, Smith N. (2024) 'Psychiatric nurse and educator perspectives on professional boundaries in nursing education: An interpretive description study', Journal of Professional Nursing, 52, pp. 80–85. https://doi.org/10.1016/j.profnurs.2024.03.011.

Torjesen I (2019) Childhood trauma doubles risk of mental health conditions. BMJ 364:l854. https://doi.org/10.1136/bmj.l854. Accessed 7 Feb 2026

University of Liverpool News (2025) People with personality disorders often use language differently… (press release). Available at: https://news.liverpool.ac.uk/2025/12/22/people-with-personality-disorders-often-use-language-differently-our-research-reveals-how/. Accessed 7 Feb 2026

Mental Health Conditions

Diagnosis Versus Formulation

There is debate across literature about whether psychiatry should replace category-based diagnosis with a psychological formation system (Seery et al. 2021).

There are currently two main classifications for mental health disorders. The International Classification of Diseases (ICD) and Diagnostic and Statistical Manual of Mental Disorders (DSM) have been around since the mid-twentieth century (First et al. 2021). Currently around 35 countries globally use the ICD-11 classification, which was ratified by the World Health Organization in 2019, including the United Kingdom (Nafarieh et al. 2025; Seemüller 2023).

Clinical formulation was introduced over 30 years ago and is a summary of a person's problems and a summary of opinion on what might go wrong in the future and what steps should be taken to improve matters (Baird et al. 2017).

Gelder (1994) in the *Concise Oxford Textbook of Psychiatry* describes formulation as:

> Concise assessment of diagnosis, aetiology, treatment and prognosis…it is not merely a summary in another form but an exercise in clinical reasoning.

Formulation should follow the following areas (Baird et al. 2017):

The Presenting Problem

This is a very brief summary of a clinical problem and the questions that need to be answered within the formulation. This should also include a summary of the concerns that are at the core of referral or assessment.

R. Bage, *Mental Health Skills for Adult Nurses & Non-Specialist Healthcare Workers*, https://doi.org/10.1007/978-3-032-32835-9_4

The History

This is the summary of what is known, and what remains unknown, about a service user's background and their key events within their life. This should not read as a narrative but instead summarise the importance and relevance of the events to the current situation. In this, it is useful to think about what may be triggers or maintainers of their current difficulties and also document any strengths or protective factors that exist. Any gaps should also be highlighted.

The Concerns

This is a summary of things that may go wrong, and what form further deterioration or crisis is likely to take. These concerns should be plausible. The emphasis should focus on those which are most likely to happen, rather than the most serious and should draw on literature (such as rates of relapse).

The Plan

This should be a clear statement of what action is proposed and what the next steps will be. This should be a patient-centred approach and the responses to the questions and concerns must be proportionate (Baird et al. 2017).

One of the key advantages of clinical case formulation is that it advocates for collaborative working in terms of their presentation and interventions. This is important as it gives service users the opportunity to highlight their strengths and hopefully gives practitioners a deeper understanding of the service user (Macneil et al. 2012).

Diagnostic Overshadowing

Happell et al. (2016) state that diagnostic overshadowing presents one possible reason for healthcare inequity. Kanne (2013) defines diagnostic overshadowing as a negative bias impacting a professional's judgement regarding co-occurring disorders in service users who have either a learning disability or a mental illness. Many of us will have encountered service users who have not felt heard, with their symptoms and underlying conditions not being fully explored or understood. Diagnostic overshadowing is explored at length with both my own adult and mental health nursing students, and should be at the forefront of all our minds when working in practice. We all carry biases, and stereotypes. People with mental health conditions and learning disabilities remain at risk of diagnostic overshadowing and it continues to be the one of the causes of death for people in the UK.

Psychosis

Reflective Questions
What do you know about psychosis?
What interactions have you had with people who have a diagnosis of psychosis?

Throughout this chapter, the ICD-11 codes for diagnosis will be included to allow practitioners to reference the ICD-11 further as needed. Table 1 shows the current ICD-11 codes for schizophrenia (WHO 2019).

The term psychosis encompasses several different symptoms associated with alterations to a person's perception, thoughts, mood and behaviour. Psychosis is a syndrome associated with the dysregulation of two different neurotransmitters—dopamine and serotonin. There is also evidence to suggest abnormal functioning of some of the body's key brain circuits in the frontal, temporal and mesostriatal brain areas (McCutcheon et al. 2020). The causes of psychotic disorders are unknown, but it does appear to involve a number of genetic, social and environmental risk factors. Identified risk factors include the following:

- Stressful life events (e.g. bereavement, job loss, relationship breakdown).
- Adverse childhood events (e.g. parental loss or abuse).
- Family heritage (studies have evidenced higher risk in south-Asian and black populations).
- Migration.
- Urban living.
- Cannabis use or other substance use.
- High-dose corticosteroid use.
- Early life factors from exposure in utero.
- Exposure to the protozoan parasite.
- Parental age (under 20, or over 40).

The 2014 Adult Psychiatric Morbidity Survey (APMS) established that the prevalence rate of people in England who had received a psychotic disorder diagnosis (schizophrenia, schizoaffective disorder, or affective psychosis) was approximately 0.5%.

Table 1 ICD codes for schizophrenia

ICD-11 code	
6A20	Schizophrenia
6A21	Schizoaffective disorder
6A22	Schizotypal disorder
6A23	Acute and transient psychotic disorder
6A24	Delusional disorder
6A25	Symptomatic manifestations of primary psychotic disorder
6C40.6	Alcohol

Table 2 Psychosis symptoms

Severe affective mood disorders with psychotic symptoms e.g. severe depression or bipolar disorder	Schizophrenia, schizoaffective disorder, or affective psychosis	Cerebrovascular disorder, cerebral tumours, or temporal lobe epilepsy
Drug—induced psychosis—caused by cannabis, corticosteroids, opioids, cocaine and amphetamines	Post-traumatic stress disorder	Obsessive compulsive disorder
Autism spectrum disorder	Communication disorders	Sepsis

Table 3 Postive vs. negative symptoms

Positive symptoms	Negative symptoms
Disorganised behaviours	Emotional blunting
Disorganised speech	Reduced speech
Thought disturbance	Loss of motivation
Delusions (fixed or falsely held beliefs)	Self-neglect
Hallucinations	Social withdrawal

Psychosis can be present in a range of disorders including those listed in Table 2 (NICE 2025):

Individuals with a psychosis disorder experience combinations of both 'positive' symptoms and 'negative' symptoms, which you can see in Table 3 (NICE 2025).

Hallucinations or Delusions?

Hallucinations affect the perception. Hallucinations should be considered as incomprehensible experiences that the person describes or interprets, and that perception is accompanied by feelings. Delusion is a false belief based on incorrect inference about external reality and its explanations are in conflict with the evidence. Delusions affect the cognition. Both of these can be an extreme cause of distress for service users (Kumari et al. 2013).

Examples of Delusions

Persecutory Delusions—this is a belief that something or someone is trying to harm you.

Grandiose Delusions—This is a belief that you have unusual or extreme abilities, power, or importance. A common grandiose delusion is a thought you are an important religious figure such as God.

Delusions of Reference—This is when there is a belief that events, objects, or actions refer specifically to them. A common delusion of reference is that the TV presenter is specifically talking to them.

Somatic Delusion—These are false beliefs about physical health or bodily functions. This might be that you have a chip inserted under your skin to control you.

Hallucinations

Hallucinations are associated with a range of medical conditions, ranging from Hashimoto's disorder to deficiencies in D and B12 vitamins and Parkinson's disorder or traumatic brain injuries (Waters and Fernyhough 2017). Hallucinations have been one hallmark of mental illness for centuries, but evidence suggests they are not always pathological in nature. How many of us have had the experience of hearing our name called aloud or hearing another's voice when there is no-one there? We may have worked with service users who have seen their dead spouse. Figures suggest that one in 6 people have seen, heard or experienced ghosts or spirits (Chaudhury, 2010). It is always important to explore the physical and mental health of people experiencing hallucinations.

Prodromal Period

Psychosis is one disorder that can be preceded by a prodromal period which can last up to 18 months. A prodromal period may present with cognitive, emotional and behavioural changes which may lead to reduced interest in daily activities or problems with sleep, memory, concentration, communication, motivation or affect. A prodromal period may also have low-intensity psychotic symptoms which may be intermittent in presentation. This may include things such as hallucinations or unusual thoughts. The prodromal period will then commonly be followed by an acute psychotic episode with hallucinations, delusions and disturbances. Prodromal periods can be hard to identify at the time.

Case Study

Aaron was found in the university library at 4 am, pacing between the aisles and muttering to himself. Security at the library reported he was whispering 'the exam knows what I am thinking' Security also stated he appeared really frightened and confused and was covering his ears.

Security has called the wellbeing services at the library and supported him to attend A + E. They had also managed to get hold of his friend at university who had met him up in the department and was able to give you some history.

Jake, Aaron's friend, told you that he is currently preparing for his final year medical exams. They report he had been getting very limited sleep, sometimes only about 2 hours. They report he also has had boxes of energy drinks delivered and is only drinking energy drinks and eating protein snacks.

He tells you that he has worked out the exam answers by 'frequencies' and the university bosses 'were after him' as he knew all the results and he was the 'cleverest person ever at the university'.

What makes you concerned about his presentation?
What triggers have Aaron had going on?
What would be your management plan for Aaron?

Management of Psychosis

One of the most important element of the management of psychosis, or at risk of psychosis is doing an assessment regarding risk to self or risk to others. Current NICE guidance recommends that people with a diagnosed psychotic disorder be offered a trial of antipsychotic medication in conjunction with family intervention, individual CBT, and art therapy (NICE 2025).

It is important to only work within your scope of knowledge when completing risk management plans. Full risk assessments should be completed by specialist mental health professionals. However, risk is an important area to understand and to include in any referrals on to services. Areas to consider or enquire about in risk:

- Do they have a history of self-harm?
- Do they have any suicidal ideation? Do they have a plan, and have they had any previous attempts?
- Do they feel hopeless?
- Do they use recreational drugs?
- Do they use alcohol?
- Do they gamble or do they have a gambling issue?
- Do they have any social support?
- Have they got any personal stressors e.g. recent hospital stay, recent relationship breakdown?
- Are they a carer? Do they look after children or other family?
- Do they have a history of confrontation or violence to others?
- Do they have access to, or history of carrying weapons? (NICE 2025)

Case Study

There are a range of concerns for Aaron which are indicating an acute mental health crisis. The first concern is a persecutory delusion, where he is stating things like 'The exam knows what I am thinking' and 'the university bosses are after me'. He is also making some grandiose delusions, in which he thinks she is someone grand or very important. There are also examples of potential thought disorders, in which he is pacing, muttering and appearing confused. There are also potential signs of auditory hallucinations, as he is covering his ears. We could take this as a sign that he is trying to block something out.

Further concern could be had because there is a significant decline in his presentation. He also appears to have no insight into his current deteriorating mental health.

The current risks could be risk to self, such as risk of paranoia, deterioration or harm through exhaustion or physical ill health. There is also some evidence of risk from others, as he thinks people may be after him. A big concern here would be the risk of self-neglect, due to his limited diet, disrupted sleep and disrupted routine.

There are a number of current triggers going on for Aaron which can be typical for this type of service user. There is a significant amount of academic stress, which is also linked to sleep deprivation. He is also not eating or drinking sufficiently. We may at this point also want to explore predisposing factors which are unknown at this point. You may want to explore substance misuse, family history of mental illness, previous episodes of ill health and previous stress responses. You may want to explore what happened in previous exam seasons or A-Levels.

If you were the clinician in A + E, your immediate concern must be the risk factors. You would want to assess, and document, his current risks (as a non-mental health professional) and try to assess his current level of insight. You would want to make an urgent mental health referral, either to liaison psychiatry or crisis services. He is likely to need a Mental Health Assessment.

If you have concerns about a person's presentation and have concerns about a person experiencing psychosis or prodromal period of psychosis, this patient will need support from a mental health team. Current NICE guidelines state that it is not advised to start antipsychotic treatment whilst awaiting specialist assessment unless under advice from a consultant psychiatrist.

In the community—When in the community, the patient needs a referral to the early intervention psychosis service (EIP) in your area. In some areas, you may be able to refer directly to this service, in others you will be required to refer through a central referral system of primary care.

In an inpatient ward—When in inpatient or A + E services, service users can be referred directly to mental health liaison services. These will be contactable by your local switchboard, and they may be available 24 hours a day.

Ongoing management of psychosis may include prescribing of medication, crisis plans, reviewing of physical health annually, and ongoing support to try and prevent relapses of their condition. It is estimated that 80% of people show response to treatment within the first year, and one in every five people has no further psychotic episodes within the next 5 years.

Depression

In the Table 4, the ICD-11 codes for depression can be seen (WHO 2026).

In the ICD-11, depression is defined as 'Depressive disorders are characterised by depressive mood (e.g. sad, irritable, empty) or loss of pleasure accompanied by

Table 4 ICD-11 code for depression

ICD-11 code	
6A70	Single episode depressive disorder
6A71	Recurrent depressive disorder
6A72	Dysthymic disorder
6A73	Mixed depressive and anxiety disorder
GA34.41	Premenstrual dysphoric disorder
6A7Y	Other specified depressive disorders
6A7Z	Depressive disorders, unspecified

other cognitive, behavioural, or neurovegetative symptoms that significantly affect the individual's ability to function. A depressive disorder should not be diagnosed in individuals who have ever experienced a manic, mixed or hypomanic episode, which would indicate the presence of a bipolar disorder'. It may also be accompanied with other symptoms such as:

- Low self-worth.
- Excessive or inappropriate guilt.
- Hopelessness.
- Recurrent thoughts of death or suicidal ideation or evidence of attempted suicide.
- Significantly disrupted sleep or excessive sleep.
- Significant changes in appetite/weight.
- Psychomotor agitation.
- Reduced energy or fatigue.

The symptoms of depression can be broadly grouped into emotional, neurovegetative and cognitive symptoms. Anxiety is common to be seen alongside depression, with approximately 2/3 of people with depression also having anxiety. A major depressive disorder is different from general unhappiness and typical feelings of sadness (Malhi and Mann 2018).

Less Severe Depression

Less severe depression encompasses subthreshold and mild depression and is typically people who score less than 16 on the PHQ-9 scale. The Patient Health Questionnaire-9 (PHQ-9) is a self-administered version of the PRIME-MD diagnostic instrument for depression (Kroenke et al. 2001).

More Severe Depression

More severe depression encompasses moderate and severe depression; this is typically people scoring more than 16 on the PHQ-9 scale.

There can be a number of different patterns of depression:

- Single episode depressive disorder (a person's first and only episode).
- Recurrent depressive disorder (at least two depressive episodes).
- Bipolar disorder.

Depression is a common mental health disorder. It is thought to impact 4% of the population worldwide, with approximately 332 million people in the world having a diagnosis of depression worldwide. Depression is more common in women than men (WHO, 2025a)

There is no single model or mechanism which can explain all aspects of the disease. Some of the key theories are the monoamine hypothesis, the hypothalamic-pituitary-adrenal axis changes or inflammation, neuroplasticity and neurogenesis, or structural or functional brain changes (Malhi and Mann 2018). The monoamine hypothesis is maybe the most commonly discussed, with research suggesting that monoamine neurotransmitters (serotonin, noradrenaline and dopamine) have a role (Malhi and Mann 2018). Twin and adoption studies have also identified that it is moderately hereditable, although specific genes have not been identified (Malhi and Mann 2018).

Depression has a range of risk factors including:

- Physical health.
- Physical inactivity.
- Harmful use of alcohol.
- Adverse life events (e.g. unemployment, bereavement, traumatic events).

Having a long-term physical health problem can increase your risk. It is thought about 40% of people with depression and anxiety have a long-term condition such as COPD or musculoskeletal disorders. Around 70% of people with medically unexplained symptoms have mental health comorbidities. Due to the structural challenges between mental health and adult services, see chapter "The Background of Physical Health and Mental Health", it can be hard for these service users to access support.

Depression also impacts a service users' ability to engage in recovery and adherence to medication. A recent study into asthma medication found that people with depressive symptoms were more prone to poor adherence and scepticisms towards medication adherence. The study found that depression had both a direct and indirect effect on adherence (Dong et al. 2024).

Treatment

The aim of treatment is to have complete remission of depressive symptoms, which can often be achieved by psychology therapy and/or psychotherapy (Malhi and Mann 2018).

For those with less severe depression, service users may choose to have active monitoring rather than accept psychological or pharmaceutical treatment. NICE guidelines (NG222) currently suggest further assessment in 2–4 weeks' time following initial assessment. Other treatment options available for those with less severe depression are:

- Guided self-help e.g. Cognitive behavioural therapy.
- Group cognitive behavioural therapy.
- Group behavioural activation.
- Individual CBT.
- Individual BA.
- Group exercise.
- Group mindfulness and meditation.
- Interpersonal psychotherapy.
- Pharmacology e.g. SSRI's.
- Counselling.
- Short-term psychodynamic psychotherapy (NICE 2022).

For those with more severe depression, there are a range of treatment options available:

- CBT and an antidepressant.
- Individual CBT.
- Individual behavioural activation.
- Antidepressant medication.
- Individual problem-solving.
- Counselling.
- Short-term psychodynamic psychotherapy.
- Interpersonal psychotherapy.
- Guided self-help.
- Group exercise (NICE 2022).

Case Study

Ivy attends the practice nurse to get her annual review. Ivy tells you it has been the first time she has gone out for 'about 9 months'. She says her son in law had brought her, but he 'wasn't very happy about it' and swore at her constantly on the way. She becomes tearful.

She says life has been really difficult for the last 18 months since her daughter, son-in-law and 3 children moved in. They said they were only going to stay for 3 or 4 weeks, but now are refusing to leave.

Ivy states she has stopped going out, seeing or ringing her friends, or doing anything much. Her daughter now uses her car, and she doesn't feel up to walking too far. Ivy says she gets by on snacky food and just stays in bed most of the time.

Ivy does not give you much eye contact throughout and instead stares at the floor. She is wearing dirty clothes, and her hair seems matted at the back. Her left lens of her glasses is missing, and the glasses are taped together.

What concerns do you have about Ivy in the case study?
What symptoms of depression are she displaying?
What would you do in this situation?

In Ivy's case, she has a number of concerns regarding her physical health, mental health and safeguarding. Ivy has reported that her son-in-law was not happy bringing her to the appointment and she reports that she is fearful of him and the home environment. She also discusses that her daughter is using the car but is not clear whether this is consensual. There is also evidence of self-neglect, with poor hygiene, nutrition and spending most of her time in bed. All of these factors may warrant a safeguarding referral.

She has significant symptoms of depression. There is evidence of social withdrawal, and loss of interest in her usual and current activities. She is tearful and has limited motivation and energy. There is evidence of helplessness and social withdrawal.

You need to prioritise a warm and therapeutic relationship. If you feel confident, you may want to use a mental health assessment tool such as the PHQ-9. You may also want to take the opportunity to do physical health assessments such as blood pressure and BMI. Ivy does need specialist support, and you may choose to refer to local community mental health team for a mental health review. Ivy may also be a good candidate for NHS Talking Therapies.

In your appointment, you may wish to develop a safety plan with Ivy and arrange further follow-up. She would benefit from a safeguarding referral. If she highlights further risks, you may refer through to Crisis Team for urgent same-day support.

Anxiety Disorders

The World Health Organization states that anxiety is the most common mental health disorder in the world (WHO 2025b).

People with an anxiety disorder may have specific fear or worry about a specific situation, for example a panic attack, or have anxiety about a broad range of everyday situations. Typically, these anxiety conditions occur over an extended period. Other symptoms may include:

- Trouble concentrating.
- Trouble making decision.
- Feeling irritable or restless.
- Experiencing nausea.
- Stomach aches or abdominal distress.
- Having heart palpitations.

- Sweating, trembling, or shaking.
- Trouble sleeping.
- Having a sense of impending danger or panic.

There are a range of anxiety disorders, which will be discussed below in more detail.

Generalised Anxiety Disorder (GAD)

Generalised anxiety is a disorder that involves persistent and excessive worry about daily activities or events for at least 6 months (WHO 2025b; BMJ 2025). Symptoms can include:

- Restlessness or nervousness.
- Being easily fatigues.
- Poor concentration.
- Irritability.
- Muscle tension.
- Sleep disturbance.
- Sweating.
- Light headedness.
- Palpitations.
- Dizziness.
- Epigastric discomfort.

The key diagnostic factors for GAD are presence of risk factors, excessive worry for at least 6 months, anxiety not confined to another mental health condition or medication/substance (BMJ 2025).

There are a number of risk factors for GAD: family history of anxiety, physical or emotional stress, history of trauma (physical, sexual, or emotional) and other anxiety disorder. Diagnosis can normally be completed through clinical diagnosis, but other tests may be necessary to rule out physical health conditions (e.g. thyroid function tests, urine drug screens, pulmonary function tests) (BMJ 2025).

Case Study

You have been seeing Magdalena for the last 9 years after she had a traumatic left leg amputation following a work incident. Magdalena has coped well and has been getting on well with her new prosthesis. She is independent in all mobility, self-care and household tasks.

Over the last 2 appointments (you see her 3 monthly) Magdalena has withdrawn and has started attending with her partner. You notice she has lost her bubbly self.

Her partner asks to speak to you alone and tells you that she keeps talking about worrying it will happen again, and feelings of worry that she can't stop.

You speak to Magdalena and she tells you that she is too worried to do anything anymore, and she is not sleeping well. Magdalena states she doesn't want to leave the house anymore, and she feels 'unsafe' in big shops and when picking up her daughter on the playground.

What aspects of trauma-informed care are relevant in this case study?
What symptoms of anxiety is Magdalena displaying?
What physical health factors would you consider with Magdalena?
What next steps would you take with Magdalena?

With Magdelena, you would want to focus on some trauma-principles. You may focus on making sure she feels safe, making sure she trusts you, and ensuring she has choice within the appointment. You would want to ensure that you notice any signs or re-emerging trauma and ask Magdelena to talk to you if she does have concern about this happening.

Magdalena is showing many signs of anxiety re-occurring. There are the psychological symptoms such as worrying that she 'can't stop' and intrusive thoughts. She is also reporting that she feels unsafe in crowds. There is evidence that she is avoiding places which she would usually have gone to. There are also physical signs such as poor sleep, hypervigilance and restlessness.

You would want to ensure you consider physical health factors in Magdelena's case. For example, you would think about her current use of her prosthesis, and how this may be impacted by her mental health and sleep. You also want to think about her current self-care, and the impact this may have on her mobility and activity levels.

Next steps are important for Magdelena. You would want to focus on giving her a safe space to talk and normalising her feelings. If you feel confident, you may want to complete a GAD-7 or similar screening tool. You want to discuss treatment plans openly with Magdelena and the options for referral on. Magdelana would be a good candidate for Talking Therapies.

Panic Disorder

Panis disorder is characterised by recurring panic attacks over at least a 1-month period (BMJ 2025). A panic attack is defined by ICD-11 (World Health Organization 2019) as a sudden increase in fear or apprehension which peaks rapidly.

Symptoms include:

- Sweating.
- Palpitations.
- Increased heart rate.
- Chest pain.

- Feelings of choking.
- Feelings of dizziness.
- Light-headedness.
- Shortness of breath.
- Fear of losing control.
- Fear of imminent death (Aslam et al. 2024).

People with a panic disorder are often concerned about having further panic attacks and may change behaviours to try and avoid having further panic attacks (BMJ 2025).

Debate exists in literature about the causes of panic attacks in panic disorder. Some argue that panic attacks are caused by biological explanations and neurochemical dysregulation (e.g. Charney et al. 1989; Klein et al. 1993). Others argue that panic attacks are caused by a cognitive misinterpretation (Clark 1986). Three core predictions are made from the cognitive theory of panic disorder:

- Misinterpretations of body sensations are more likely to be witnessed in panic service users than those who do not experience panic attacks (Clark et al. 1985).
- Panic and/or anxiety should increase in panic service users if conditions activate catastrophic misinterpretations (Clark et al. 1985).
- Reducing these catastrophic misinterpretations of bodily sensations should reduce the panic attacks in panic service users (Clark et al. 1985).

Salkovskis (1991) suggests a further predication:

- Service users with panic engage in safety-seeking behaviours which therefore maintain the panic disorder. This prevents individual with a panic disorder from benefitting from a disconfirmatory experience (Salkovskis 1991; Salkovskis et al. 1999).

Risk Factors

There are a number of risk factors that relate to panic disorder; these include:

- History of first-degree relatives having panic disorders.
- Female.
- Being between 18 and 39 years.
- White or Native American ethnicity.

Diagnosis can normally be identified by clinical assessment and presence of risk factors, unexpected onset, apprehension and worry and behavioural avoidance (BMJ 2025). It may be necessary to order further investigations such as ECG, blood glucose, thyroid function tests and metabolic panels (BMJ 2025).

NICE suggests psychological treatment, medication and self-help all have roles to play in successfully treating panic disorder (NICE 2020), and will be explored in more detail.

Psychological Treatment

Cognitive behavioural therapy is the offered treatment for panic disorder and will normally be offered between 7 and 14 hours of treatment. The treatment is normally considered finished after no longer than 4 months (NICE 2020).

Medication

There are a number of different options for panic disorder. These are normally antidepressants such as selective serotonin reuptake inhibitors (SSRI's) or tricyclic antidepressants (NICE 2020).

Self Help

Self-help is also an option to support service users to reduce panic attacks. This could range from support groups, advice on exercise or self-help programmes (NICE 2020).

Social Anxiety Disorder

Social anxiety disorder is a disorder characterised by an excessive fear of social and performance events where a person is afraid of being negatively evaluated or rejected by others (BMJ 2025).

Social anxiety disorder is one of the most common disorders, with high risk for comorbidity with other conditions, such as anxiety, depression and substance misuse. It often causes impairments in daily functioning, reduced quality of life, increased difficulty in forming relationships, and impaired school and work performances (BMJ 2025). Key diagnostic factors include presence of risk factors, anticipatory anxiety and worry, tachycardia and hyperventilation (BMJ 2025).

There are a number of risk factors:

- Psychiatric comorbidities (e.g. anxiety, mood disorders, substance-misuse disorders).
- Genetic predisposition.
- Temperamental factors.
- Parenting styles.

Breathing Exercises and Grounding Techniques

Breathwork comprises various different practices which encompass regulating the way that one breathes, in order to support mental, emotional and physical health (Oxford English Dictionary 2019). There are multiple different breathing exercises with complex historical roots such as yoga, Tibetan Buddhism, and psychedelic communities (Fincham et al. 2023). Breathing exercises can be easily taught, and learned in group settings, which make them very effective treatments that can be offered at scale (Fincham et al. 2023).

Case Study

Karol attends the wellbeing service at college reporting that he has started to feel so anxious about being in college that he cannot go to his lectures anymore, and he becomes so panicked in case he is asked to talk in a seminar. Karol says his attendance has dropped to 46% and he is worried he will get 'kicked out'.

Karol says he has always been an introvert and shy, but the symptoms have worsened since he had a new lecturer who started setting group presentations. Her says he is worried that people will judge him as English is not his first language. He says he goes red and feels sick in sessions, and he is embarrassed.

Karol also talks about his ruminating thoughts, which means he is struggling to switch off at night after he has done a presentation. Karol says he doesn't feel particularly anxious anywhere else and still likes going outdoors with his friends.

What symptoms of social phobia does Karol have?
What physical symptoms is he displaying?
What strategies could you use to build rapport with Karol?
What interventions may support Karol in the short and medium terms?

Diagnosis can be through clinical diagnosis, but investigations could be ordered to rule out other conditions (e.g. blood glucose, serum thyroid-stimulating hormone, and a toxicology screen) (BMJ 2025).

Karol has a number of symptoms of social phobia which include:

- Fear of being judged.
- Avoidance behaviours.
- Avoidance of situations where he may need to present.
- Ruminating thoughts.

There are also a number of physical symptoms that Karol is presenting such as blushing, nausea, panic symptoms, poor sleep and struggling to switch off, and shakiness. This might describe a fight vs. flight response going on with Karol.

The important thing with Karol is to ensure that he has a safe space to discuss his concerns with you, and to ensure that you reinforce that anxiety in social situations is common and treatable. You may also want to approach some of the cultural elements of this by checking that he is happy to talk in his second language to you. You may want to focus on active-listening and avoid using directive communication with him. A good approach here to use is a strengths-based approach, where you are focussing on what he is doing well.

Psychoeducation is an important tool for Karol and making sure he has some resources to take away. You might want to print him off some resources about breathing and grounding techniques. You may want to help Karol identify some triggers at this appointment, or you may leave that until a later point. Karol would be a good candidate for Talking Therapies.

Agoraphobia

Agoraphobia is when somebody feels anxiety in public places, or fear when leaving a "safe place". Others with agoraphobia may fear being left alone (called monophobia) or dislike feeling trapped in an environment (Anxiety UK, n.d.). Agoraphobia is treated under the same NICE guidelines as other anxiety disorders.

Post-traumatic Stress Disorder

Post-traumatic Stress Disorder (PTSD) is a condition estimated to have affected 3.9% of the world population at some point in their life (WHO 2024). Whilst the majority of people worldwide will experience something potentially traumatic during their lifetime, only a minority will go on to develop a PTSD. PTSD rates are higher after some specific traumatic events—violence, conflict or war and sexual violence (Kessler et al. 2017; Koenen et al. 2017; Charlson et al. 2019).

PTSD was first included in the DSM-III in 1980 and has been known by many names such as 'shell shock', 'Vietnam syndrome', and 'battered woman syndrome'. Much of the early work about PTSD relates to military contexts, but PTSD is experienced by many more people than those just in combat (Billings and Nicholls 2025).

Symptoms of PTSD, seen in Table 5, can be separated into two categories—re-experiencing symptoms and avoidance symptoms (PTSDUK 2025):

Complex PTSD is a subset of PTSD. It is a newly separate diagnosis in the ICD-11 (Billings and Nicholls 2025). It arises after exposure to an event or series of events of an extremely threatening or horrific nature, commonly prolonged or repetitive events of a threatening or horrific nature. These are often prolonged or repetitive events from which escape is challenging or impossible (e.g. torture, slavery, genocide campaigns, prolonged domestic violence or repeated abuse). C-PTSD is characterised by the core symptoms of PTSD as mentioned above, but also can include:

- Severe problems in affect regulation.
- Persistent beliefs about self as diminished or defeated.
- Deep feelings of shame, guilt or failure related to traumatic event.
- Persistent difficulties in sustaining relationships (NICE 2018).

Table 5 Symptoms of PTSD

Re-experience symptoms	Avoidance symptoms
Flashbacks	Staying away from places or events that might be reminders of the experience
Re-occurring memories	Feeling that you need to keep yourself busy
Distressing and intrusive thoughts or images	Using alcohol or drugs to avoid memories
Physical sensations—sweating, trembling, pain, feeling sick	Feeling emotionally numb or cut off
Hyperarousal	Being unable to remember details of the trauma
	Emotional numbing

Treatment for Children

Treatment for children often involved individual trauma-focussed CBT interventions. This is typically provided over 6–12 sessions by trained practitioners. The trauma-focussed CBT intervention will involve elaboration and processing of trauma memories, processing of trauma-related—emotions and provide psychoeducation about reactions to trauma (NICE). Eye movement de-sensitisation and reprocessing (EMDR) can also be considered if they do not engage or respond effectively to trauma-focussed CBT (NICE).

Treatment for Adults

Treatment for adults includes trauma-focussed CBT intervention including cognitive processing therapy, cognitive therapy for PTSD, narrative exposure therapy and prolonged exposure therapy. Adults should be offered 8–12 sessions, psychoeducation, elaboration and processing of trauma memories, processing of trauma-related emotions and focus on re-establishing adaptive functioning. EMDR can also be considered for non-combat related trauma if the service user prefers this. Service users can also be offered trauma-focussed computerised CBT (NICE). Pharmaceutical treatment may also be offered to adults with PTSD, and this will be explored further in chapter "Healthcare Environments". Treatment for complex PTSD is a little vaguer. NICE suggest increasing the duration or number of therapy sessions (NICE 2018).

Personality Disorders

Reflective Questions

What do you know about personality disorders already?

What have you heard in clinical practice about personality disorders?

What do you want to know about working more effectively with those with a personality disorder diagnosis?

Personality disorder is characterised by problems in functioning of aspects of self (e.g. self-worth, identity), and/or interpersonal dysfunction that have persisted over an extended period of time (over 2 years). The disturbance causes patterns of cognition, emotional experience, emotional expression and maladaptive behaviours across personal and social situations. The disturbance is associated with substantial distress or impairment in personal, family, social, educational, occupational or other areas of functioning (ICD, 11).

Essential features include:

- Enduring disturbance characterised by problems in aspects of self-and/or interpersonal dysfunction.
- The disturbance has persisted over an extended period of time (e.g. 2 years or more).
- Disturbance manifests in patterns of cognition, emotional experience, emotional expression, and or behaviour that are maladaptive.
- Manifests across a range of personal and social situations (not limited to specific relationships or social roles).
- Symptoms are not due to direct effects of medication or substances, including withdrawal effects. Symptoms are not better accounted for by another mental disorder, nervous system disorder, or another medical condition.
- Disturbance is associated with substantial distress or significant impairment in personal, family, social, educational, occupational or other important areas of functioning.
- Personality disorder should not be diagnosed if patterns of behaviour are developmentally appropriate (e.g. independent self-identity in adolescence) (ICD, 11).

Personality diagnosis changed in the most recent ICD publication. Personality disorder has become one unitary syndrome, characterised by core interpersonal dysfunction and a range of other traits (NHS Digital n.d.). Previous diagnosis, and diagnosis with the DSM-5-TR, sees personality diagnosis separated into ten categories:

- Paranoid.
- Schizoid.
- Schizotypal.
- Antisocial.
- Borderline.
- Histrionic.
- Narcisstic.
- Avoidant.
- Dependent.
- Obsessive–compulsive.

Current ICD-11 diagnosis sees personality disorder separated into four subcategories—mild, moderate, severe, severity unspecified.

6D10.0 Mild Personality Disorder

- Disturbances affect some areas of functioning of the self but not others or affect all areas but are of mild severity.
- Some challenges with interpersonal relationships or in performance in expected occupational and social roles. Some relationships are maintained or roles fulfilled.
- Mild manifestations of personality disturbances (e.g. individuals' sense of self may be somewhat contradictory or inconsistent to how others view them).
- Can be associated with substantial distress or with impairment in personal, family, social, educational, occupational, or other areas of functioning.

6D10.1 Moderate Personality Disorder

- Disturbances affect multiple areas of functioning to the self (e.g. stability and coherence of identity).
- Marked problems in most interpersonal relationships and the performance of most expected social and occupational roles are compromised to some degree.
- Relationships characterised by conflict, avoidance, withdrawal, or extreme dependency.
- Manifestations of personality disturbances are generally of moderate severity (e.g considerable difficulty maintaining positive self-esteem).
- Sometimes associated with harm to self or others.
- Impairment in personal, family, social, educational, occupational or other important areas of functioning.

6D10.2 Severe Personality Disorder

- Severe disturbances in functioning of the self.
- Problems in interpersonal functioning which affect almost all relationships.
- Severe disturbances in multiple areas of functioning of the self (e.g. sense of self may be so unstable that individuals report not having a sense of who they are or so rigid that they refuse to participate in any but an extremely narrow range of situations).
- Problems in interpersonal functioning seriously affect virtually all relationships and the ability and willingness to perform expected social and occupational roles are severely compromised or absent.
- Specific manifestations of personality disturbance are severe.
- Severe Personality Disorder is often associated with harm to self or others.
- Severe Personality Disorder is associated with severe impairment in all or nearly all areas of life, including personal, family, social, educational, occupational, and other important areas of functioning.

6D10.Z Personality Disorder, Severity Unspecified

There is no medication that can treat any of the personality disorders. There is huge variation in presentation, and treatment and management must be person-centred and involve the service user. NICE guidelines vary by diagnosis, but focus on psychological therapies to allow people to manage and treat the disorder (NICE, 2025). NICE guidelines state that people with borderline personality disorder should not be excluded from any health or social care service because of their diagnosis or because they have self-harmed (2009). Personality disorders remain some of the most stigmatised areas of mental health, as well as some of the most misunderstood health conditions.

There are a group of service users who have been told that there is something 'wrong' with their personality. As discussed by Keir Harding, this is a label given to those who have survived abuse. It is thought that, at least. 90% of people given an emaotionally unstable personality disorder diagnosis have survived abuse (Harding, 2025). When working with service users with thjs diagnosis, please consider the consequences and emotions of such a diagnosis and remember the principles of trauma informed care.

Bipolar Disorder

Please see the ICD codes for bipolar disorder below in Table 6 (WHO 2026).

Bipolar disorder is a chronic psychiatric condition which is characterised by recurrent episodes of mania and depression. These disorders are known to contribute significantly to disability and mortality and linked to suicide and cardiovascular disease. Bipolar disorders have significant genetic, neurobiological and environmental factors and are often accompanied by comorbidities (Oliva et al. 2025).

Symptoms for bipolar include:

- Increased self-esteem or grandiosity.
- Decreased need for sleep.
- Racing thoughts.
- Compulsion to keep talking.
- Flight of ideas.
- High distractibility.
- Increased goal-directed activity.
- Excessive involvement in activities with potential losses (e.g. spending lots of money) (Jain and Mitra 2023).

Table 6 Bipolar disorder ICD 11 Codes

ICD-11	
6A60	Bipolar type 1 disorder
6A61	Bipolar type 2 disorder
6A62	Cyclothymic disorder
6A6Y	Other specified bipolar or related disorders
6A6Z	Bipolar or related disorders, unspecified

What do we mean by flight of ideas?

Flight of ideas is a thought disorder which references the expression of rapidly shifting thoughts in an individual. These thoughts will be expressed through language. When talking to someone with flight of ideas, their speech may become incomprehensible, as the ideas are fluttering between ideas so quickly (Gaag 2013; Bertschy et al. 2020).

Listening to someone with flight of ideas is unforgettable. They will be moving through ideas and thoughts so quickly that you struggle to follow any kind of theme of conversation.

Type One Bipolar

The criteria for this are met when there has been at least one manic episode, which might have been preceded or followed by a hypomanic episode or major depressive episode (Jain and Mitra 2023).

Type Two Bipolar

This criterion is met when there has been at least one current or past hypomanic episode and a major depressive episode. There will have been no manic episode.

Pharmacological treatments are a key factor in bipolar treatment. Lithium is the medication which is current first-line within the UK for bipolar disorder. If lithium is not tolerated well, service users may consider an antipsychotic as a second line choice. There are more details of this in the pharmacological chapter (NICE 2025).

Dementia and Delirium

Dementia is characterised by impairment in two or more cognitive domains relative to that expected given the individual's age and general level of cognitive functioning. This represents a decline from the service user's previous level of functioning. Memory impairment is a key element in most forms of dementia, but cognitive impairment is not restricted to memory (ICD-11).

The ICD-11 codes for dementia are included in Table 7 below (ICD-11 2026).

There are over 200 different types of dementia established, and the most common will be covered in more detail below (Harrison Dening 2023).

Alzheimer's Disease

Alzheimer's disease is a chronic and progressive neurodegenerative disorder.It is characterised by general cognitive decline, memory loss, and impaired

Table 7 ICD codes for dementia

ICD-11	
6D80	Dementia due to Alzheimer disease
6D80.0	Dementia due to Alzheimer disease with early onset
6D80.1	Dementia due to Alzheimer disease with late onset
6D80.2	Alzheimer disease dementia, mixed type, with cerebrovascular disease
6D80.3	Alzheimer disease dementia, mixed type, with other nonvascular aetiologies
6D80.Z	Dementia due to Alzheimer disease, onset unknown or unspecified
6D81	Dementia due to cerebrovascular disease
6D82	Dementia due to Lewy body disease
6D83	Frontotemporal dementia
6D84	Dementia due to psychoactive substances including medications
6D84.0	Dementia due to use of alcohol
6D84.1	Dementia due to use of sedatives, hypnotic or anxiolytics
6D84.2	Dementia due to use of volatile inhalants
6D84.Y	Dementia due to other specified psychoactive substance
6D85	Dementia due to diseases classified elsewhere
6D85.0	Dementia due to Parkinson disease
6D85.1	Dementia due to Huntington disease
6D85.2	Dementia due to exposure to heavy metals and other toxins
6D85.3	Dementia due to human immunodeficiency virus
6D85.4	Dementia due to multiple sclerosis
6D85.5	Dementia due to prion disease
6D85.6	Dementia due to normal pressure hydrocephalus
6D85.7	Dementia due to injury to the head
6D85.8	Dementia due to pellagra
6D85.9	Dementia due to down syndrome
6D85.Y	Dementia due to other specified diseases classified elsewhere

reasoning. Alzheimer's is the leading cause of dementia in older adults (Safiri et al. 2024). It has a complicated etiology with factors including genetics, the environment, and ageing. There are a number of hypotheses in play, such as cholinergic, amyloid, tau protein, inflammatory, oxidative stress, metal ion, glutamate excitotoxicity, microbiota-gut-brain axis, and abnormal autophagy (Zhang et al. 2024). The risk of Alzheimer's disease and other types of dementia increases with age, affecting an estimated 1 in 14 people over the age of 65 and 1 in every 6 people over the age of 80 (NHS 2024)

Vascular Dementia

The pathobiology of vascular dementia is significantly linked with the ageing process. Key risk factors include age, diet, obesity, hypertension, hypercholesterolaemia, alcohol abuse, diabetes, smoking, air pollution and physical inactivity (Morgan and Mc Auley 2024). There is opportunity to reduce risks of vascular dementia with appropriate management of type 2 diabetes and hypertension (Morgan and Mc Auley 2024).

Frontotemporal Dementia

Frontotemporal dementia is a neurogenerative disease and accounts for approximately 10% of middle-age-onset dementias. Initial characterisation is selective degeneration of frontal and/or temporal lobe, which leads to changes in behaviour, speech disorders and psychiatric symptoms (Antonioni et al. 2023).

Dementia with Lewy Bodies

Dementia with Lewy bodies is the leading cause of late-life dementia and is often underdiagnosed. Clinical sensitivity for dementia with Lewy Bodies is low, and it has significant morbidity and mortality (Fullam et al. 2026; Price et al. 2017). There is a significant disparity between the number of cases diagnosed clinically and those diagnosed via neuropathology at postmortem. It has a worse prognosis than Alzheimer's dementia, with a faster cognitive impairment (Prasad et al. 2022). The most common complaint is memory dysfunction, followed by visual hallucinations, depression, problem-solving abilities, gait disturbances and tremor and stiffness (Auning et al. 2011).

Alcohol-Related Brain Damage

Wernicke–Korsakoff syndrome and Wernicke's encephalopathy are potentially reversible neurological disorders caused by a deficiency in or severe depletion of thiamine. This can result from chronic alcoholism, poor nutrition, long-term parenteral feeding or bariatric surgery (Zahr et al. 2011). Signs of Wernicke's encephalopathy include uncontrollable and jerky eye movements, problems walking and co-ordination, confusion and memory loss. Immediate medical attention should be sought for this, and anyone undergoing a planned alcohol withdrawal programme will be treated in advance for these complications (NICE 2017).

One of biggest ethical debates in dementia (or delirium) care is around the moral debate of whether it is acceptable to provide misleading reassurance to a service user. An example of this may be "don't worry, you are just visiting'. A report copiled by the Mental Health Foundation titled 'What is Truth' looked at truth and lying in dementia care. It was the report's view that perceiving different realities and beliefs only as symptoms of dementia, while occasionally appropriate, is not sufficient to address the range of complex experiences people living with dementia. The panel agreed five terms that encompass types of caring interventions and responses to people living with dementia experiencing different realities and beliefs (Mental Health Foundation 2016). These were

1. Whole truth telling.
2. Looking for alternative meaning.
3. Distracting.
4. Going along with.
5. Lying.

The report clarifies that, as clinicans, we should start from the position of 'whole truth telling'. When/if this is causing distress, we should then move to a truth that may contain an untruth (Mental Health Foundation 2016).

Delirium

Delirium is characterised by disturbance of attention, orientation and awareness that develops within a short period of time, presenting as significant confusion of global neurocognitive impairment, with transient symptoms that may fluctuate depending on underlying cause or aetiology. Delirium often causes disturbance of behaviours and emotions and may include impairment in multiple cognitive domains (WHO 2026). The ICD-11 codes for delirium are included in Table 8.

At times, it can be challenging to identify the differences between dementia and delirium, especially when working directly in clinical practice. Table 9 offers a useful table to identify the differences in presentation between the two conditions, although we must remember that often those with dementia may present with delirium as well (Jandu et al. 2026).

Management of Delirium

The management of delirium means that most people should be admitted to hospital for urgent assessment. This decision should be made based on clinical and social situation, and also by consulting family members and carers (NICE 2023).

Table 8 ICD codes for delirium

ICD-11	
6D70	Delirium
6D70.0	Delirium due to disease classified elsewhere
6D70.1	Delirium due to psychoactive substances including medications
6D70.2	Delirium due to multiple etiological factors
6D70.Y	Delirium, other specified cause
6D70Z	Delirium, unspecified of unknown cause

Table 9 The differences between delirium and dementia

Feature	Dementia	Delirium
Onset	Gradual Develops over months to years	Sudden, develops over hours to weeks
Course	Progressive and typically irreversible—normally a steady decline, although some dementias have more sudden declines	Fluctuating throughout day Often reversible with treatment
Primary Cause	Neurogenerative or vascular	Acute illness Infection Medication Dehydration Metabolic
Attention	Usually preserved until later stage	Impaired early
Memory	Short—term memory loss is common and progressive	May be impaired Likely to fluctuate
Level of consciousness	Typically, normal until later stages	Often reduced or fluctuating
Hallucinations	Possible—common in Lewy Body	Common—often visual
Reversibility	Generally irreversible	Often reversible
Progression	Slow, steady decline in most cases.	Rapid changes
Treatment Focus	Symptom management, support	Treating underlying cause

Management in primary care should only be considered if all of the following are present:

1. The benefits of management in primary care outweigh the benefits of hospital admission, or the person is clinically well enough to stay at home.
2. The symptoms of delirium are not harmful to the person or others and can be managed safely in primary care.
3. The cause of delirium is known and treatable.
4. The person can receive constant supervision and care from a healthcare professional trained in the management of delirium—to minimise complications.
5. Close clinical follow-up can be arranged (NICE 2023).

Reflective Questions

Which presentation do you see most in your service?

Key Learning Points

Adult nurses and other practitioners will often see poor mental health before a mental health diagnosis is made. Early recognition is key, and you might be the first person to have a conversation with a service user about their mental health. It is important that you feel confident in this.

Every practitioner should feel some confidence in assessing basic mental health skills such as mood, self-harm and suicidal ideation, sleep, cognitive changes and substance misuse. These are important observations and assessments to then make referrals onwards.

You do not need specialist knowledge, and nobody is expecting you to become fully fledged mental health nurses. However, the skills to understand how symptoms may group together and reflect on whether something bigger is going on are important.

Never forget the importance of interprofessional practice—and always endeavour to work together. We can learn so much more if we work together.

Conclusion

This chapter has explored a broad range of mental health conditions, providing readers with the knowledge and clinical awareness required to support service users that they work with.

Discussion around psychosis, depression, anxiety disorders, trauma-related conditions, personality disorders, bipolar disorder and neurocognitive disorders helped to highlight how each condition varies. Case studies throughout the chapter illustrate how theoretical knowledge translates into practice, and you have opportunity to return to these case studies as your knowledge and reflections develop.

This chapter discusses the importance of practitioners listening and learning with service users. Working with those who have a mental health diagnosis requires empathy, reflective practice and strong interprofessional communication. As we progress through the principles explored in the book, practitioners will be able to reflect further on their own practices, experiences and reflections which shape person-centred care.

References

Antonioni A, Raho EM, Lopriore P, Pace AP, Latino RR, Assogna M, Mancuso M, Gragnaniello D, Granieri E, Pugliatti M, Di Lorenzo F, Koch G (2023) Frontotemporal dementia, where do we stand? A narrative review. Int J Mole Sci 24(14):11732. https://doi.org/10.3390/ijms241411732. Accessed 7 Feb 2026

Anxiety UK (n.d.) Agoraphobia. Available at: https://www.anxietyuk.org.uk/anxiety-type/agoraphobia/ Accessed: 22 July 2026

Aslam SY, Zortea T, Salkovskis P (2024) The cognitive theory of panic disorder: a systematic narrative review. Clin Psychol Rev 113:102483. https://doi.org/10.1016/j.cpr.2024.102483. Accessed 7 Feb 2026

Auning E, Rongve A, Fladby T, Booij J, Hortobágyi T, Siepel FJ, Ballard C, Aarsland D (2011) Early and presenting symptoms of dementia with Lewy bodies. Dement Geriatr Cogn Disord 32(3):202–208

Baird J, Hyslop A, Macfie M, Stocks R, Van der Kleij T (2017) Clinical formulation: where it came from, what it is and why it matters. BJPsych Adv 23(2):95–103. https://doi.org/10.1192/apt.bp.115.014670. Accessed 7 Feb 2026

Bertschy G, Weibel S, Giersch A, Weiner L (2020) Racing and crowded thoughts in mood disorders: A data-oriented theoretical reappraisal. L'Encéphale 46(3):202–208

Billings J, Nicholls H (2025) PTSD and complex PTSD, current treatments and debates: a review of reviews. Br Med Bull 156(1). https://doi.org/10.1093/bmb/ldaf015. Accessed 7 Feb 2026

BMJ Best Practice (2025) Generalised anxiety disorder, panic disorder and social anxiety disorder: clinical guidance. Available at: https://bestpractice.bmj.com/. Accessed 7 May 2026

Charlson F, van Ommeren M, Flaxman A, Cornett J, Whiteford H, Saxena S (2019) New WHO prevalence estimates of mental disorders in conflict settings: a systematic review and meta-analysis. Lancet 394(10194):240–248. https://doi.org/10.1016/s0140-6736(19)30934-1. Accessed 7 Feb 2026

Charney DS, Woods SW, Heninger GR (1989) Noradrenergic function in generalized anxiety disorder: effects of yohimbine in healthy subjects and patients with generalized anxiety disorder. Psychiatry Res 27(2):173–182. https://doi.org/10.1016/0165-1781(89)90132-7. Accessed 7 Feb 2026

Chaudhury S (2010) Hallucinations: Clinical aspects and management. Ind Psychiatry J 19(1):5–12. https://doi.org/10.4103/0972-6748.77625. Accessed 22 July 2026

Clark DM (1986) A cognitive approach to panic. Behav Res Ther 24(4):461–470. Accessed 15 August 2025

Clark DM, Salkovskis PM, Chalkley AJ (1985) Respiratory control as a treatment for panic attacks. J Behav Ther Exp Psychiatry 16(1):23–30. https://doi.org/10.1016/0005-7916(85)90026-6. Accessed 7 Feb 2026

Dong R, Sun S, Sun Y, Wang Y, Zhang X (2024) The association of depressive symptoms and medication adherence in asthma patients: the mediation effect of medication beliefs'. Res Soc Adm Pharm 20(3):335–344. https://doi.org/10.1016/j.sapharm.2023.12.002. Accessed 7 Feb 2026

Fincham GW, Kartar A, Uthaug MV, Anderson B, Embere Hall L, Nagai Y, Critchley H, Colasanti A (2023) High ventilation breathwork practices: an overview of their effects, mechanisms, and considerations for clinical applications. Neurosci Biobehav Rev 155. https://doi.org/10.31234/osf.io/z62fv. Accessed 7 Feb 2026

First MB, Gaebel W, Maj M, Stein DJ, Kogan CS, Saunders JB, Poznyak VB, Gureje O, Lewis-Fernández R, Maercker A, Brewin CR, Cloitre M, Claudino A, Pike KM, Baird G, Skuse D, Krueger RB, Briken P, Burke JD, Lochman JE, Evans SC, Woods DW, Reed GM (2021) An organizationand category-level comparison of diagnostic requirements for mental disorders in ICD-11 and DSM-5. World Psychiatry 20(1):34–51.

Fullam S, Harrison JR, Anderson KN, Fearon C, O'Connor A, Taylor J-P, O'Dowd S (2026) Dementia with Lewy bodies: a practical guide to clinical diagnosis and management. Pract. Neurol. 26(1):4–16

Gelder M (1994) Concise Oxford textbook of psychiatry. Oxford University Press, Oxford

Happell B, Ewart SB, Platania-Phung C, Stanton R (2016) Participative mental health consumer research for improving physical health care: an integrative review. Int J Ment Health Nurs 25(5):399–408. https://doi.org/10.1111/inm.12226. Accessed 7 Feb 2026

Harding K (2025) The painful consequences of personality disorder diagnosis. The Guardian, 24 January. Available at: https://www.theguardian.com/society/2025/jan/24/the-painful-consequences-of-personality-disorder-diagnosis. Accessed 22 July 2026

Harrison Dening K (2023) Dementia 1: types, risk factors, and recognising signs and symptoms. Nurs Times 119(3). Available at: https://www.nursingtimes.net/clinical-archive/dementia/dementia-1-types-risk-factors-and-recognising-signs-and-symptoms-27-02-2023/. Accessed 7 May 2026

Jain A, Mitra P (2023) Bipolar Disorder. StatPearls Publishing. https://www.ncbi.nlm.nih.gov/books/NBK558998/. Accessed 12 Jul 2026

Jandu JS, Mohanaselvan A, Fang X (2026) Differentiating delirium versus dementia in older adults. [Updated 2025 Feb 17]. In: StatPearls [Internet]. StatPearls Publishing, Treasure Island. Available from: https://www.ncbi.nlm.nih.gov/books/NBK570594/. Accessed 7 May 2026

Kanne S (2013) Diagnostic overshadowing. In: Volkmar FR (ed) Encyclopedia of autism Spectrum disorders. Springer, New York. https://doi.org/10.1007/978-1-4419-1698-3_398. Accessed 7 May 2026

Kessler RC, Aguilar-Gaxiola S, Alonso J, Benjet C, Bromet EJ, Cardoso G, Degenhardt L, de Girolamo G, Dinolova RV, Ferry F, Florescu S, Gureje O, Haro JM, Huang Y, Karam EG, Kawakami N, Lee S, Lepine JP, Levinson D, Navarro-Mateu F, Pennell BE, Piazza M, Posada-Villa J, Scott KM, Stein DJ, Ten Have M, Torres Y, Viana MC, Petukhova MV, Sampson NA, Zaslavsky AM, Koenen KC (2017) Trauma and PTSD in the WHO world mental health surveys. Eur J Psychotraumatol 8(sup5):1353383. https://doi.org/10.1080/20008198.2017.1353383. Accessed 7 May 2026

Klein GA, Orasanu J, Calderwood R, Zsambok CE (eds) (1993) Decision making in action: models and methods. Ablex Publishing

Koenen KC, Ratanatharathorn A, Ng L, McLaughlin KA, Bromet EJ, Stein DJ, Karam EG, Ruscio AM, Benjet C, Scott K, Atwoli L, Petukhova M, Lim CCW, Aguilar-Gaxiola S, Al-Hamzawi A, Alonso J, Bunting B, Ciutan M, de Girolamo G, Degenhardt L, Gureje O, Haro JM, Huang Y, Kawakami N, Lee S, Navarro-Mateu F, Pennell BE, Piazza M, Sampson N, Ten Have M, Torres Y, Viana MC, Williams D, Xavier M, Kessler RC (2017) Posttraumatic stress disorder in the World Mental Health Surveys. Psychol Med 47(13):2260–2274. https://doi.org/10.1017/S0033291717000708. Accessed 7 May 2026

Kroenke K, Spitzer RL, Williams JB (2001) The PHQ-9: validity of a brief depression severity measure. J Gen Intern Med 16(9):606–613. https://doi.org/10.1046/j.1525-1497.2001.016009606.x. Accessed 22 July 2026

Kumari R, Chaudhury S, Kumar S (2013) Dimensions of hallucinations and delusions in affective and nonaffective illnesses. ISRN psychiatry. 616304. https://doi.org/10.1155/2013/616304. Accessed 22 July 2026

Macneil CA, Hasty MK, Conus P, Berk M (2012) Is diagnosis enough to guide interventions in mental health? Using case formulation in clinical practice. BMC Medicine 10:Art 111. https://doi.org/10.1186/1741-7015-10-111. Accessed 7 May 2026

Malhi GS, Mann JJ (2018) Depression. Lancet 392(10161):2299–2312. https://doi.org/10.1016/S0140-6736(18)31948-2. Accessed 7 May 2026

McCutcheon RA, Krystal JH, Howes OD (2020) Dopamine and glutamate in schizophrenia: biology, symptoms and treatment. World Psychiatry 19(1):15–33

Mental Health Foundation (2016) What is truth? An inquiry about truth and lying in dementia care. London: Mental Health Foundation. Available at: https://www.mentalhealth.org.uk/sites/default/files/2022-09/MHF-dementia-truth-inquiry-report.pdf. Accessed: 22 July 2026

Morgan AE, Mc Auley MT (2024) Vascular dementia: From pathobiology to emerging perspectives. Ageing Res Rev 96:102278

Nafarieh K, Krüger S, Deutscher K, Schreiter S, Mundt AP, Jung A, Fazel S, Heinz A, Gutwinski S (2025) The prevalence of prolonged grief disorder according to the international classification of diseases 11: a scoping review. Eur Arch Psychiatry Clin Neurosci. Advance online publication. https://doi.org/10.1007/s00406-025-02046-4. Accessed 7 May 2026

NHS Digital (n.d.) ICD-11 personality disorder structure. Accessed 12 Feb 2025

NHS (2024) Alzheimer's disease. Available at: https://www.nhs.uk/conditions/alzheimers-disease/. Accessed 22 July 2026

National Institute for Health and Care Excellence (NICE) (2015) Personality disorders: borderline and antisocial (QS88) Available at: https://www.nice.org.uk/guidance/qs88/chapter/quality-statement-2-psychological-therapies-borderline-personality-disorder. Accessed: 24 July 2026

National Institute for Health and Care Excellence (NICE) (2017) Alcohol-use disorders: diagnosis and management of physical complications: Recommendations (CG100). Available at: https://www.nice.org.uk/guidance/cg100/chapter/recommendations. Accessed 25 Feb 2026

NICE (2018) Post-traumatic stress disorder: evidence reviews and guidelines. NICE, London. Accessed 19 Nov 2025

National Institute for Health and Care Excellence (NICE) (2018) Borderline personality disorder: recognition and management (CG97). Available at: https://www.nice.org.uk/guidance/cg78/chapter/Recommendations. Accessed: 24 July 2026

NICE (2020) panic disorder: clinical guidance. NICE, London. Accessed 18 September 2025.

National Institute for Health and Care Excellence (NICE) (2022) Depression in adults: treatment and management (NG222). Available at: https://www.nice.org.uk/guidance/ng222. Accessed 12 Jan 2026

National Institute for Health and Care Excellence (NICE) (2023) Delirium: prevention, diagnosis and management (CG103). Available at: https://www.nice.org.uk/guidance/cg103. Accessed 19 Jan 2026

NICE (2025) Psychosis: assessment and management guidelines. NICE, London. Accessed 19 Sept 2025.

Oliva V, Fico G, De Prisco M, Gonda X, Rosa AR, Vieta E (2025) Bipolar disorders: an update on critical aspects. Lancet Reg Health - Eur 48:101135. https://doi.org/10.1016/j.lanepe.2024.101135.

Oxford English Dictionary (2019) Definition of breathwork

Prasad S, Katta MR, Abhishek S, Sridhar R, Valisekka SS, Hameed M, Kaur J, Walia N (2022) Recent advances in Lewy body dementia: a comprehensive review. Disease-a-Month 69(5):101441. https://doi.org/10.1016/j.disamonth.2022.101441. Accessed 7 May 2026

Price A, Farooq R, Yuan J-M, Menon VB, Cardinal RN, O'Brien JT (2017) Mortality in dementia with Lewy bodies compared with Alzheimer's dementia: a retrospective naturalistic cohort study. BMJ Open 7(11):e017504.

PTSD UK (2025) PTSD symptoms and information. Available at: https://www.ptsduk.org. Accessed 18 Feb 2026.

Safiri S, Ghaffari Jolfayi A, Fazlollahi A, Morsali S, Sarkesh A, Daei Sorkhabi A, Golabi B, Aletaha R, Motlagh Asghari K, Hamidi S, Mousavi SE, Jamalkhani S, Karamzad N, Shamekh A, Mohammadinasab R, Sullman MJM, Şahin F and Kolahi A-A (2024) Alzheimer's disease: a comprehensive review of epidemiology, risk factors, symptoms diagnosis, management, caregiving, advanced treatments and associated challenges. Front. Med. 11:1474043. https://doi.org/10.3389/fmed.2024.1474043. Accessed 22 July 2026.

Salkovskis PM (1991) The importance of behaviour in the maintenance of anxiety and panic: a cognitive account. Behav Psychother 19(1):6–19. https://doi.org/10.1017/s0141347300011472. Accessed 7 May 2026

Salkovskis PM, Clark DM, Hackmann A, Wells A, Gelder MG (1999) An experimental investigation of the role of safety-seeking behaviours in the maintenance of panic disorder with agoraphobia. Behav Res Ther 37(6):559–574. https://doi.org/10.1016/s0005-7967(98)00153-3. Accessed 7 May 2026

Seemüller F (2023) ICD-11 and mental disorders: important changes, controversies, and future directions. BMC Psychiatry 23(1). https://doi.org/10.1186/s12888-023-05186-w. Accessed 7 Feb 2026

Seery C, Bramham J, O'Connor C (2021) Effects of a psychiatric diagnosis vs a clinical formulation on lay attitudes to people with psychosis. Psychosis 13(4):1–12. https://doi.org/10.1080/17522439.2021.1901302. Accessed 7 May 2026

Gaag JVDR (2013) Flight of ideas. In: Volkmar FR (ed) Encyclopedia of autism spectrum disorders. Springer, New York. https://doi.org/10.1007/978-1-4419-1698-3_50. Accessed 7 Feb 2026

Waters F, Fernyhough C (2017) Hallucinations: a systematic review of points of similarity and difference across diagnostic classes. Schizophr Bull 43(1):32–43. https://doi.org/10.1093/schbul/sbw132. Accessed 7 May 2026

World Health Organization (2019) ICD-11 clinical descriptions and diagnostic requirements Available from: https://www.who.int/publications/i/item/9789240077263 Accessed 9 Oct 2025

World Health Organization (2024) Global PTSD statistics Available from: https://www.who.int/news-room/fact-sheets/detail/post-traumatic-stress-disorder Accessed 19 Feb 2026

World Health Organization (WHO) (2025a) Depressive disorder (depression). Available at: https://www.who.int/news-room/fact-sheets/detail/depression. Accessed: 22 July 2026
World Health Organization (2025b) Generalised anxiety disorder: diagnostic guidelines Available from: https://www.who.int/news-room/fact-sheets/detail/anxiety-disorders Accessed 19 Feb 2026
Zahr NM, Kaufman KL, Harper CG (2011) Clinical and pathological features of alcohol-related brain damage. Nat Rev Neurol 7(5):284–294
Zhang J, Zhang Y, Wang J, Xia Y, Zhang J, Chen L (2024) Recent advances in Alzheimer's disease: mechanisms, clinical trials and new drug development strategies. Signal Transduction and Targeted Therapy 9, Article 211. Available at: https://doi.org/10.1038/s41392-024-01911-3 Accessed 22 July 2026

Mental Health Through the Lifespan

Child & Adolescent

Reflective Questions

What are your concerns in working with this cohort of people?

What do you think are the biggest factors on our mental health of children and young people?

Most child and adolescent (CAMHS) specialists come from the field of mental health practice, but very little of a mental health nursing degree or similar focusses on children and young people (Baldwin 2019). In reality, much of a mental health nursing course focusses on mental health very neatly between the ages of 18–65. My own institution has recently introduced a six-week module looking specifically at child and adolescent mental health practice for mental health and child student nurses, but this is a rare opportunity. However, childhood is the very bedrock of the future, and we should not underestimate the importance of child and adolescent mental health.

The 2022 Mental health of Children and Young People (MHCYP) survey looked into the mental health of children and young people aged 7–24 years living in England. This survey was also completed in 2017, 2020 and 2021. Eighteen percentage of 7- to 16-year-olds had a probable mental health disorder. Eleven to Sixteen-year-olds with a probable mental health disorder were less likely to feel safe at school. Additionally, they are less likely to enjoy learning (NHS Digital 2022).

Bronfenbrenner's Ecological Theory of Human Development (Vélez-Agosto et al. 2017)

Bronfenbrenner's ecological theory conceptualised children's development as a process of bi-directional and reciprocal relationships between a developing individual and those in their environment (such as parents or teachers within the microsystem) (Bronfenbrenner 1979). Bronfenbrenner was a Russian-born American

R. Bage, *Mental Health Skills for Adult Nurses & Non-Specialist Healthcare Workers*, https://doi.org/10.1007/978-3-032-32835-9_5

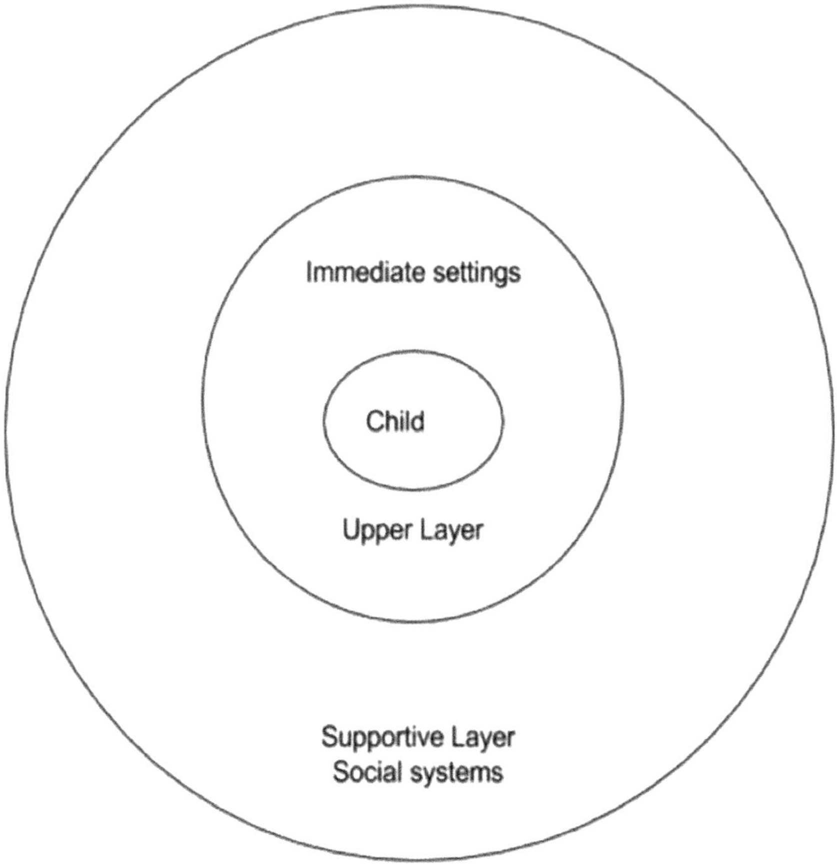

Fig. 1 Ecological model (Velez-Agosto et al. 2017)

psychologist who studied human development (Tong and Shidong An 2024). In Fig. 1, you can see version one of the models developed in 1974. In Fig. 2, you can see the later version published in 1977 (Vélez-Agosto et al. 2017). The model provides a very visual tool to help explain relationships within environments and people.

Bronfenbrenner's framework consists of four levels (Vélez-Agosto et al. 2017):

The 'individual' level—this would be the child
Microsystem—this is the children's immediate relationships that develop with families and teachers
Mesosystem—this is where the children interact with local communities
Exosystem—this involved the social systems and neighbours
Macrosystem—this consists of the influences from culture and media, and the relationship on how this impacts the children's developments (Velez-Agosto et al. 2017).

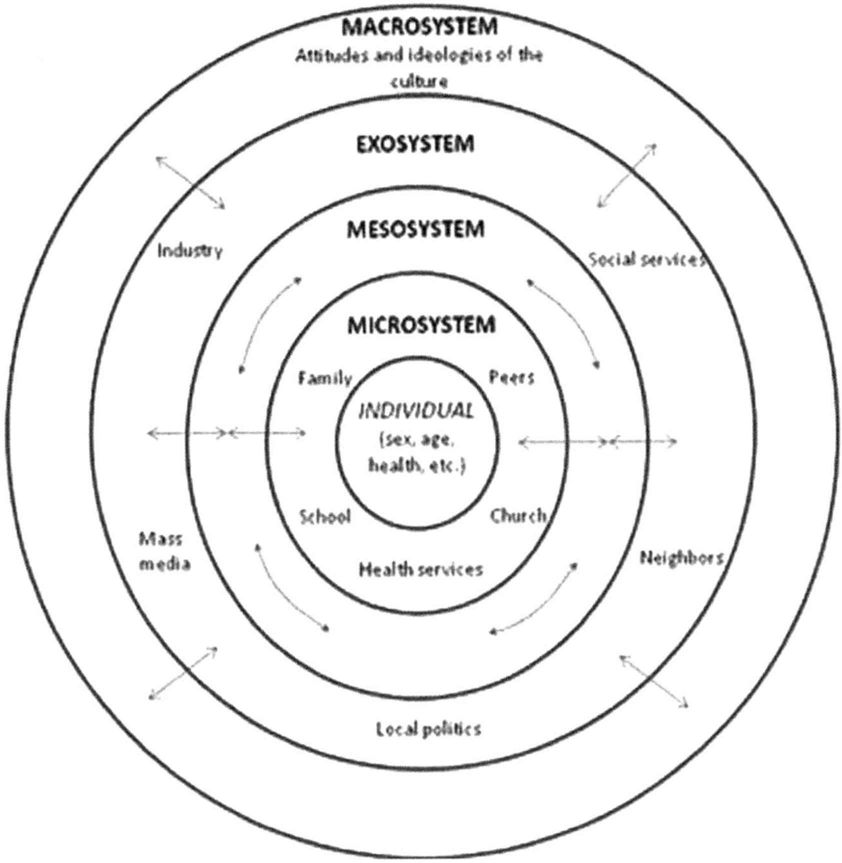

Fig. 2 The ecological theory of human development

Adverse Childhood Experiences

Adverse childhood experiences (ACEs) are one of the leading reasons to physical illness and mental health difficulties worldwide (Deneault et al. 2025). Through varied mechanisms, including neurodevelopmental disruption, reprogramming of stress receptors and epigenetic changes, experiencing ACEs increases risk of cognitive challenge, lifelong diseases, premature mortality, psychopathology and adulthood social problems (Madigan et al. 2023). ACEs are a risk factor to later mental health illness across the spectrum (Rienecke et al. 2022).

A 2010 cross-sectional survey completed in 2010 found 44.6% of childhood-onset disorders and 25.9 to 32% of later-onset disorders took root in ACEs (Green et al. 2010). A later meta-analysis and systematic review found that those with at least four ACEs were at increased risk of all health outcomes compared to those with no ACEs. Associations were strong for sexual risk-taking, mental ill-health and

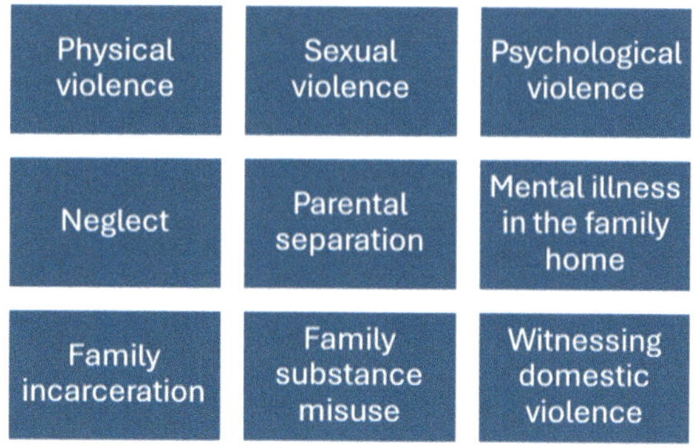

Fig. 3 Examples of ACE's

problematic alcohol use and strongest for drug use and interpersonal and self-directed violence (Hughes et al. 2017).

ACE's include things that impact children directly, such as abuse or neglect. Other ACE's affect children through their living environments such as parental conflicts, substance abuse or mental ill-health (Hughes et al. 2017). Some examples of ACE's are included in Fig. 3.

Schooling

One Australian study found that children with experience of adverse childhood experiences have higher rates of being suspended from school (Bell et al. 2021).

Evidence suggests that for students within two-parent households in England, absences from school are a significant contributor to experiencing poor mental health. The effect of this is amplified further if there are other vulnerabilities such as Education, health and Care (EHC) plans or any type of SEND or are eligible for free school meals. Equally, poor mental health is also correlated to a child's absence from school (ONS 2025).

A 2022 research study found that nearly half of young people in England state that school is not an enjoyable experience but instead consider it something they need to 'get through'. Stressors included being required to learn subjects of little interest to them, the pressure of needing to make difficult decisions and the emphasis on attainment in exams (McPherson et al. 2023). Young people also described feeling unsupported by teaching staff in their schools, with higher levels of this amongst those with SEND or from backgrounds of socioeconomic disadvantage (McPherson et al. 2023).

Since 2019, mental health support teams (MHSTs) have worked with schools and colleges across England. As of early 2025, 600 of these teams are operational and approximately 52% of teachers and learners have access to these services (NHS England 2025). These teams are made up of clinical lead practitioner and educational mental health practitioners who have had specialist training to support young people (LPFT, n.d).

THRIVE

The THRIVE model is a nationally used in service development (Farr et al. 2021). The thrive model is a needs-based model and focusses on ideas such as shared decision making (Wolpert et al. 2019). It has been designed for:

- Children and young people aged 0–25.
- Families and carers of children and young people.
- Professional who seeks awareness with wellbeing needs or those at risk of mental health difficulties.

It is an integrated and person-centred approach, which focusses on a need-led approach to delivering mental health services for young people and their families. It was developed by specialists and authors from the Anna Freud National Centre for Children and Families, and colleagues from the Tavistock and Portman NHS Foundation Trust (Wolpert et al. 2019).

The THRIVE framework guides systems by summarising the needs of children and young people into five groups:

- Getting advice.
- Getting risk support.
- Getting help.
- Getting More help.
- Thriving (Wolpert et al. 2019).

The national i-THRIVE Programme (NIP) helps child and adolescent sites in adopting the key principles of THRIVE. I-THRIVE was created following implementation guidelines to support wider adoption of THRIVE principles of child and adolescent mental health services (Moore et al. 2023).

Sippy et al. (2025) completed a study of experiences of staff using i-THRIVE to assess effectiveness and local system working relationships impact on the progress of i-THRIVE. They used a quasi-experimental design across 10 implementation and 10 comparison sites. The results suggest implementation staff sites were more likely to report using THRIVE and more knowledgeable of the basic principles of THRIVE. Interestingly, sites with highly effective working relationships showed increased improvement in 'THRIVE-like' features. The findings of this study suggest there is importance of working relationship effectiveness in adoption and implementation of multi-agency policies such as i-THRIVE.

Adults

The mental health of the working-age adults appears to be deteriorating across the UK. The greatest increase in poor mental health has been in the younger-age groups of 16- to 34-year-old people. The evidence suggests that people with lower-level qualifications, those unemployed and people living in the North of England are at higher risk (The Health Foundation 2025).

The world is also a complex place. A recent mental health survey found that 82% of people feel anxious about major issues like war and conflict (MIND 2025). In my own practice, I have seen people come in to see mental health professionals after arguments about politics, BREXIT and other political and societal events. A barometer of any society should be the health and wellbeing of the communities that it makes up. However, in the UK, only a minority of people are living with high levels of positive mental health and collective mental health is deteriorating (Mental Health Foundation 2017).

There has been a growing body of work that argues that our increasing knowledge about mental health is influencing diagnosis. Foulkes and Andrews (2023) argue two clear points. Firstly, mental health awareness efforts are leading to more accurate reports which can only be viewed as a positive step. Secondly, they argue that awareness efforts are leading the interpretation of milder forms of distress as mental health problems. This can lead to over-labelling of normal changes in our emotion as a mental health condition.

Work

Work is considered beneficial to health and wellbeing (Khan and Boardman 2017). Equally, the cost of people being out of work due to mental health is estimated at £30 billion in the UK alone. People with work-limiting mental health conditions are half as likely to be in work than those with no health conditions (The Health Foundation 2025).

In late December 2025, an estimated 957,000 people were not in employment, education or training (NEET) which is 12.8% of all 16- to 24-year-olds. Being a 'NEET' is strongly related to poorer outcomes for individuals over their lifetime including lower earnings and worse health. Increased reporting of ill health among young people since 2015 is driven primarily by mental health and neurodevelopmental conditions (The Health Foundation 2026).

Good working environments can contribute by providing:

- A livelihood.
- Monetary reward.
- A sense of confidence.
- Purpose.
- Achievement.
- An opportunity for positive relationships and inclusion in a community.
- Social contacts.
- Routine (Khan and Boardman 2017; WHO 2024).

Poor working conditions risk causing stress and can lead to mental health disorder, and unemployment is a risk for suicide (Minshall et al. 2024). A survey commissioned by the Royal College of Psychiatrists found that 9% of adults had to take time off work due to mental ill-health in the last year, and 6% stated that somebody in their household had to.

University

It is a similar picture in universities. The proportion of young people who disclosed a mental health condition to their university has increased from 1% in 2010/11 to nearly 6% in 2022/23 (Lewis and Stiebahl 2025). Studies have found some of the reasons for the decline in mental health include academic performance, self-esteem, pressure to succeed, body image and friends (Emmerton et al. 2024).

Abrahart Versus University of Bristol (Equality and Human Rights Commission 2024a)

Natasha Abrahart, from Nottingham, was studying physics at the University of Bristol. Natasha ended her life on the day she was due to give a presentation in a 329-seat lecture theatre, after being diagnosed with chronic social anxiety disorder in February 2018 (BBC News 2016). The university had considered making reasonable adjustments for Natasha and examining her through a different method. However, it had not taken steps to do so, or to discuss this with her. University of Bristol said Natasha had failed to engage with its Disabled Students Service, which would assess what reasonable adjustments to put in place. It also argued that the method of assessment – an oral assessment – was a competence standard and therefore outside the parameters of the Equality Act 2010 (Equality and Human Rights Commission 2024b). A judge ruled the university had breached its duties under the Equality Act by failing to make "reasonable adjustments" for Natasha in light of her debilitating anxiety (BBC News 2016) In this court case, the judge found there is 'no statute or precedent' concerning a duty of care owed by a university to a student to take reasonable steps to avoid and not to cause injury and harm.

The University Mental Health Charter was published in 2019 and provides a set of evidence-informed principles to support universities to adopt a whole-university approach to mental health and wellbeing (Hughes and Spanner 2019). The framework is composed of 18 themes and mapped against 4 domains which are summarised below (Hughes and Spanner 2019).

Learn

- Transition into university.
- Learning, teaching and assessment.
- Progression.

Support

- Support services.
- Risk.
- External partnerships and pathways.
- Information sharing.

Work

- Staff Wellbeing.
- Staff development.

Live

- Proactive interventions and a mentally healthy environment.
- Residential accommodation.
- Social integration and belonging.
- Physical environment (Hughes and Spanner 2019).

Parenthood

Research conducted in Australia found that 23.3% of all children in Australia have a parent with a non-substance mental illness. Just over 20% of mental health service users have dependent children and 14% of participants reported having at least one parent with a mental illness (Maybery et al. 2009). Figures in the UK look similar, with around 1 in 3 children reporting living with a parent with an emotional distress. Figures suggest 1 in 4 children lived with a mother reporting symptoms of emotional distress and 1 in 8 living with a father reporting symptoms of emotional distress (PHE 2020).

A 2025 study suggests that within the perinatal period, many parents experience mental health difficulties including OCD, postpartum psychosis and psychotic-like experiences (Foreman et al. 2026).

Cost of Living

Many of the adults today have lived through many financial crises across the globe. In recent memory, we have the financial crash, Ukraine War and multiple middle east crises, all of which have pushed up the cost of living across the glove.

60% of UK residents report that the cost-of-living crisis is negatively impacting their mental health, with a further 23% stating they are having problems sleeping because of their concerns about rising costs (Lawson et al. 2023).

Older Adults

It is expected that by 2030, one in six people across the world will be over the age of 60 (WHO 2025a). Research suggests that wellbeing and health are closely linked, more so than working-aged adults (Steptoe et al. 2015). Research from across the globe has shown that older people are often stereotyped as ill, dependent or incompetent (Swift et al. 2017; RCPsych 2018). Older adult services in mental health have typically started at age 65. This is despite the national pension age in the United Kingdom being 66 years old. In 2024, figures suggested that 15% of adults between the age of 65–74 had a mental health condition, compared to 3% of those 75–84 and 2% of those 85 + (Centre for Ageing Better 2023). Research has demonstrated that age bias is visible in a number of health conditions, including transient ischaemic attacks, minor

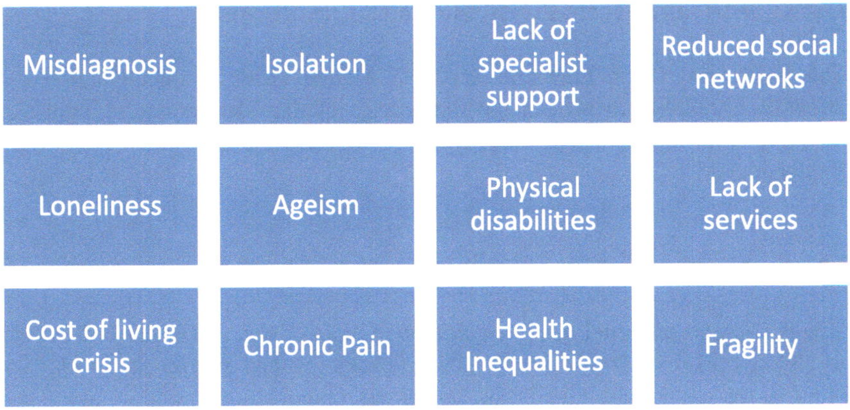

Fig. 4 Older adult risk factors for poor mental health

strokes and the under use of mental health services (Fairhead and Rothwell 2006; Centre for Policy on Ageing 2009). There is evidence that some groups of older adults have higher risk of mental health difficulties than others. There are several risk factors for older people's mental health included in Fig. 4 (Iskander-Reynolds 2024).

Residential Care and Care Homes

There are high levels of depression and acute mental and neurological illness in older residents (Iskander-Reynolds 2024). A systematic review completed in 2015 found that generalised anxiety disorders and specific phobias were the most common anxiety disorders in older adults (Creighton et al. 2015).

Poverty

Relative pensioner poverty is at the highest rate this century, and 2.1 million pensioners in the UK have an income that is less than 60% of the national average, More than one million older people are thought to have no savings, and two million older adults in the UK are living in rented accommodation (Centre for Ageing Better 2023). People who are in poverty and more likely to be in 'less than good health' than people who are not in poverty (The Health Foundation 2025). People with poor finances have made choices such as delaying retirement, socialising less, and cutting back on social activities due to the cost of living (Age UK).

Living with Long-Term Physical Health Conditions

The NHS Long Term Plan and the NHS Mental Health Implementation Plan 2019/20–2023/24 both set out the importance of the NHS providing consistent access to the mental health care for older adults with functional needs (NHS England, 2025).

Loneliness

Social isolation and loneliness are common in older adults, and the two often coexist (Bandyopadhyay 2024). WHO (2025b) estimates that approximately 11.8% of older adults experience loneliness. Loneliness could be described as a social or emotional experience resulting from a lack of meaningful relationships (Bandyopadhyay 2024).

Frailty

Frailty is a long-term health condition that reflects the increased vulnerability to adverse health outcomes. It is a spectrum disorder (British Geriatrics Society 2025). Frailty is common, with more than one in ten people over 65 having frailty. This figure increases to over 50% of those in hospital or in a care home (British Geriatrics Society 2025).

Community Mental Health Framework

The Community Mental Health Framework (NHS England 2019) offers a vision for how adult and older adult mental health services will be delivered. Within this, older adult services are discussed regards the need for integration into wider systems of support for those living with neurodegenerative and frailty conditions or living in care homes (Iskander-Reynolds 2024). We will explore this further in a later chapter.

Transitions

Transitions can often be a highly traumatic period for service users and their families (Cowan 2025). Transition is an important aspect of the delivery of mental health services, and RCPsych suggest that there should be clear protocols and frameworks for transition between services (RCPsych 2019). Transitions can affect all service users differently, and can be particularly challenging in those with a personality disorder where there has been history of poor attachment or relationships. Many transitions in mental health may be planned months to years in advance - it is crucial to make the transitions transparent and planned wherever possible.

Many young people have experienced a poor continuity of care within the transition period from CAMHS services to Adult Mental Health Services (AMHS) (Rethink 2024). For the vast majority of service users, CAMHS to AMHS transitions are poorly planned, executed and experienced (Singh et al. 2010). Equally, transitions across child to adult service in any speciality can be difficult. These transitions are known to fail to meet the needs of the young people and families at time of change and can lead to deterioration in health or disengagement from services (Sipanoun et al. 2024).

The 'On Your Own Feet Ahead' theoretical framework was developed in the Netherlands in 2008, and has eight key elements of good healthcare transition care for those moving between paediatric and adult services and which is divided into three core categories (van Staa et al. 2020):

1. Interventions to improve the organisation of care.
2. Interventions to stimulate independence and self-management of adolescents.
3. Collaboration with young people (and their families) and within the multidisciplinary team of professionals, working both in paediatric care and adult care (van Staa et al. 2020).

Key Learning Points

It is important to remember that mental health shifts across the lifespan—we are all on a dynamic and influenced by factors such as biology, social roles, environmental factors and transitions. We must remember to consider all of these factors when assessing our service users.

Mental health challenges are impacted by factors that are happening socially around us. This might include war, finances, education and cost of living crises. We must remember that mental health can easily be influenced by factors that we are all living through.

The things that happen in our childhood will impact us for the rest of our lives. It is always important to ensure we are working in a trauma-informed way.

Transitions between services are hard. If you are working within a service where there are transitions, please remember to plan this well. We all play an important role in preparing, co-ordinating and advocating for our service users within transition periods.

When working with older adults, please remember that this group is influenced by many social and health factors, such as loneliness, frailty and poverty.

Conclusion

Mental health is impacted by complex webs of biological, psychological and social factors that change throughout our lifespan. However, these periods do not happen in isolation and are influenced by what has gone before. Childhood and adolescence form a real foundation to our future life, and any adverse childhood effects experienced will continue to impact our wellbeing, functioning and vulnerability to mental ill-health. The evidence we have seen in this chapter shows very clearly the value of trauma-informed practitioners and the importance of early intervention and prevention in reducing long-term difficulties. Early support, positive relationships and stable environments can play a significant role in promoting resilience and improving future mental health outcomes. Practitioners therefore have a responsibility not only to respond to distress, but also to recognise opportunities for prevention and health promotion at the earliest stages possible.

Adulthood continues to cause challenges. Many of us will balance working life, education, parenthood and pressures such as bereavements, social relationships and financial pressures. We need to understand the importance of employment, financial stability and social relationships on ourselves and those that we support. There is a real value in ensuring we build our own support systems and helping our service users build on their own skills. In addition, adulthood can often involve periods of transition and uncertainty, such as career changes, caring responsibilities or changes in physical health, all of which may influence emotional wellbeing and coping abilities. Supporting individuals to develop resilience, coping strategies and meaningful social connections remains an important aspect of mental health care during this stage of life.

Older age brings its own challenges, including frailty, loneliness, poverty and ageism. Even with students I am surprised at how few want to work within older adult services once qualified. These, and other factors, can increase our vulnerability whilst also leading to risks around diagnostic overshadowing or lack of support. This chapter again discusses the importance of person-centred and holistic assessment and support. It is also important to recognise the strengths, experiences and resilience many older adults possess, ensuring that care does not focus solely on decline or dependency. Promoting dignity, autonomy and social inclusion should remain central to care provision for older adults experiencing mental health difficulties.

Throughout this chapter, you have had an opportunity to utilise reflective questions and case studies to build on your knowledge and skill set. By understanding the developmental, social and system perspectives, we can ensure we provide compassionate and person-centred care at whatever point of a person's life. Recognising the interconnected nature of mental health across the lifespan allows practitioners to deliver care that is empathetic, informed and responsive to the unique experiences and needs of every individual.

References

Baldwin L (ed.) (2019) Nursing Skills for Children and Young People's Mental Health. Cham: Springer. Available at: https://doi.org/10.1007/978-3-030-18679-1.

Bandyopadhyay S (2024) Loneliness and depression in older adults: living well in older age. Medicine 52(9):719–724.

BBC News (2016) Parents welcome Parliament debate on student welfare Available at: https://www.bbc.co.uk/news/articles/c0r41jdkq9jo. Accessed 22 July 2026

Bell MF, Glauert R, Ohan JL, Preen DB, Bayliss DM (2021) Early school suspensions for children with adverse childhood experiences (ACEs). J Appl Dev Psychol 76:101300. https://doi.org/10.1016/j.appdev.2021.101300. Accessed 7 May 2026

British Geriatrics Society (2025) Frailty. London: British Geriatrics Society. Available at: https://www.bgs.org.uk/sites/default/files/content/attachment/2025-02-25/BGS%20Frailty%20Briefing%20-%20Feb%202025.pdf. Accessed 11 June 2026

Bronfenbrenner U (1979) The Ecology of Human Development: Experiments by Nature and Design. Cambridge, MA: Harvard University Press.

Centre for Ageing Better (2023) State of Ageing 2023–24: Summary report. London: Centre for Ageing Better. Available at: https://ageing-better.org.uk/sites/default/files/2023-12/The-State-of-Ageing-interactive-summary-2023-4.pdf. Accessed 21 Feb 2026

Centre for Policy on Ageing (2009) Ageism and age discrimination in primary and community health care in the United Kingdom: A review from the literature. London: Centre for Policy on Ageing. Available at: http://www.cpa.org.uk/information/reviews/CPA-ageism_and_age_discrimination_in_primary_and_community_health_care-report.pdf. Accessed 16 May 2026

Cowan H (2025) Transitions of care are often traumatic for patients and must be improved. BMJ 389:r650.

Creighton AS, Davison TE, Kissane DW (2016) The prevalence of anxiety among older adults in nursing homes and other residential aged care facilities: a systematic review. Int J Geriatr Psychiatry 31(6):555–566.

Deneault A-A, Laquerre D, Beaulieu L, Myre G, Racine N, Madigan S (2025) Prevalence and correlates of adverse childhood experiences in fathers: a systematic review and meta-analysis, Child Abuse & Neglect 169(2):107651.

Emmerton RW, Camilleri C, Sammut S (2024) Continued deterioration in university student mental health: Inevitable decline or skirting around the deeper problems?, Journal of Affective Disorders Reports, 15, Article 100691.

Equality and Human Rights Commission (2024a) Advice note for the higher education sector from the legal case of University of Bristol vs Abrahart. Available at: https://www.equalityhumanrights.com/guidance/advice-note-higher-education-sector-legal-case-university-bristol-vs-abrahart. Accessed: 22 July 2026

Equality and Human Rights Commission (2024b) University of Bristol v Abrahart: equality watchdog responds to judgment in landmark case. Available at: https://www.equalityhumanrights.com/university-bristol-v-abrahart-equality-watchdog-responds-judgment-landmark-case. Accessed 21 July 2026

Fairhead JF, Rothwell PM (2006) Underinvestigation and undertreatment of carotid disease in elderly patients with transient ischaemic attack and stroke: Comparative population based study. BMJ 333(7567):525–527.

Farr J, Moore A, Bruffell H, Hayes J, Rae JP, Cooper M (2021) The impact of a needs-based model of care on accessibility and quality of care within children's mental health services: A qualitative investigation of the UK i-THRIVE Programme. Child Care Health Dev 47(4):442–450. https://doi.org/10.1111/cch.12855. Accessed 10 Dec 2025

Foreman I, Hunt T, Peterkin J and Hodgekins J (2026) Postnatal intrusive thoughts and psychotic-like experiences: exploring associations with parenting experiences and mental health. Community Ment Health J 62(3):494–512. https://doi.org/10.1007/s10597-025-01543-z.

Foulkes L, Andrews JL (2023) Are mental health awareness efforts contributing to the rise in reported mental health problems? A call to test the prevalence inflation hypothesis. New Ideas Psychol 69:101010.

Green JG, McLaughlin KA, Berglund PA, Gruber MJ, Sampson NA, Zaslavsky AM, Kessler RC (2010) Childhood adversities and adult psychopathology in the National Comorbidity Survey Replication (NCS-R) I: Associations with first onset of DSM-IV disorders. Arch Gen Psychiatry 67(2):113–123.

Hughes G, Spanner L (2019) The university mental health charter. Student Minds, Leeds. Accessed 25 August 2025

Hughes K, Bellis MA, Hardcastle KA, Sethi D, Butchart A, Mikton C, Jones L, Dunne MP (2017) The effect of multiple adverse childhood experiences on health: a systematic review and meta-analysis. The Lancet Public Health 2(8):e356–e366

Iskander-Reynolds, A. (2024) Mental health in later life: understanding needs, policies and services in England. London: Centre for Mental Health. Available at: https://www.centreformentalhealth.org.uk/wp-content/uploads/2024/03/CentreforMH_MentalHealthInLaterLife-1.pdf. Accessed 19 Dec 2025

Khan M, Boardman J (2017) Employment and mental health. OP101. London: Royal College of Psychiatrists. Available at: https://www.rcpsych.ac.uk/docs/default-source/mental-health/work-and-mental-health-library/op101-final.pdf. Accessed 12 May 2026

Lawson G, Haggar T, Hewlett K, Hall S, Piggott H, Hesketh R, Regan Z, Wojciechowska M, Dacombe R, Morgan C (2023) Experiencing the cost-of-living crisis: the impact on mental health. https://www.kcl.ac.uk/csmh/assets/esrc-csmh-cost-of-living-crisis-and-mental-health-report.pdf. Accessed 7 May 2026

Lewis J and Stiebahl S (2025) Student mental health in England: Statistics, policy, and guidance (Research Briefing CBP-8593). London: House of Commons Library. Available at: https://commonslibrary.parliament.uk/research-briefings/cbp-8593/. Accessed 11 Nov 2025

LPFT (n.d.) Mental Health Support Teams (MHST): Lincolnshire young minds. Available at: https://www.lpft.nhs.uk/young-people/lincolnshire/parents-and-carers/support-services/mental-health-support-teams. Accessed 7 May 2026

Madigan S, Cyr C, Eirich R, Fearon RMP, Ly A, Rash CL, Poole JC, Alink LRA (2023) Adverse childhood experiences: a meta-analysis of prevalence and moderators among half a million adults in 206 studies. World Psychiatry 22(3):463–471

Maybery DJ, Reupert AE, Patrick K, Goodyear M, Crase L (2009) Prevalence of parental mental illness in Australian families. Psychiatr Bull 33(1):22–26. https://doi.org/10.1192/pb.bp.107.018861. Accessed 7 May 2026

Mind (2025) The big mental health report 2025. London: Mind. Available at: https://www.mind.org.uk/media/zianu2rn/mind_the-big-mental-health-report_digital4.pdf. Accessed 11 Jan 2026

Minshall D, Tracy DK, Tarn M, Greenberg N (2024) Mental health at work: societal, economic and health imperatives align; it's time to act. Br J Psychiatr 224(4):115–116. https://doi.org/10.1192/bjp.2024.3. Accessed 7 May 2026

Moore A, Lindley Baron-Cohen K, Simes E, Chen S, Fonagy P (2023) A protocol for a multi-site cohort study to evaluate child and adolescent mental health service transformation in England using the i-THRIVE model. PLOS ONE 18(5):e0265782. https://doi.org/10.1371/journal.pone. 0265782. Accessed 12 Jan 2026

McPherson C, Bayrakdar S, Gerwitz S, Laczik A, Maguire M, Newton O, O'Brien S, Weavers A, Winch C, Wolf A (2023) Schools for all? Young people's experiences of alienation in the English secondary school system. Available at: https://www.edge.co.uk/documents/346/DD0940_-_Young_Futures_Young_Lives_FINAL.pdf. Accessed 12 Dec 2025

Mental Health Foundation (2017) Surviving or thriving? The state of the UK's mental health. Mental Health Foundation. Available at: https://www.mentalhealth.org.uk/sites/default/files/2022-06/surviving-or-thriving-state-uk-mental-health-publication.pdf. Accessed 7 May 2026

NHS Digital (2022) Mental health of children and young people in England 2022 – wave 3 follow up to the 2017 survey. NHS Digital. Available at: https://digital.nhs.uk/data-and-information/publications/statistical/mental-health-of-children-and-young-people-in-england/2022-follow-up-to-the-2017-survey. Accessed 7 May 2026

NHS England (2019) The Community Mental Health Framework for Adults and Older Adults. London: NHS England. Available at: https://www.rcpsych.ac.uk/docs/default-source/improving-care/nccmh/community-mental-health-framework-for-adults-and-older-adults.pdf. Accessed 18 Aug 2025

NHS England (2025) Mental health support in schools and colleges. Available at: https://www.england.nhs.uk/mental-health/cyp/trailblazers/. Accessed 12 Oct 2025

ONS (2025) Child mental ill health and absence from school, England. Ons.gov.uk. Available at: https://www.ons.gov.uk/peoplepopulationandcommunity/healthandsocialcare/childhealth/articles/childmentalillhealthandabsencefromschoolengland/2021to2022. Accessed 7 May 2026

Public Health England (2020) Children living with parents in emotional distress: March 2020 update. Available at: https://www.gov.uk/government/statistics/children-living-with-parents-in-emotional-distress-march-2020-update. Accessed 10 Dec 2025

Royal College of Psychiatrists (2018) Suffering in silence: Age inequality in older people's mental health care (College Report CR221). London: Royal College of Psychiatrists. Available at: https://www.rcpsych.ac.uk/docs/default-source/improving-care/better-mh-policy/college-reports/college-report-cr221.pdf. Accessed 8 Nov 2025

Royal College of Psychiatrists (2019) Bridges not walls: Good practice guidance for transitions from child and adolescent to adult mental health services (College Report CR218). London: Royal College of Psychiatrists. Available at: https://www.rcpsych.ac.uk/docs/default-source/improving-care/better-mh-policy/college-reports/cr218.pdf. Accessed 9 Oct 2025

Rethink (2024) Falling through the cracks: why young people struggle to transition to adult mental health services. Available at: https://rethink.org/news-and-stories/news-and-views/2024/falling-through-the-cracks-why-young-people-struggle-to-transition-to-adult-mental-health-services/. Accessed 21 June 2025

Rienecke RD, Johnson C, Le Grange D, Manwaring J, Mehler PS, Duffy A, McClanahan S, Blalock DV (2022) Adverse childhood experiences among adults with eating disorders: comparison to a nationally representative sample and identification of trauma profiles, Journal of Eating Disorders, 10, Article 72. Accessed 12 May 2025

Singh SP, Paul M, Ford T, Kramer T, Weaver T, McLaren S, Hovish K, Islam Z, Belling R, White S (2010) Process, outcome and experience of transition from child to adult mental healthcare: multiperspective study. Br J Psychiatry 197(4):305–312

Sipanoun P, Aldiss S, Porter L, Morgan S, Powell E, Gibson F (2024) Transition of young people from children's into adults' services: what works for whom and in what circumstances—protocol for a realist synthesis. BMJ Open 14(1):e076649. https://doi.org/10.1136/bmjopen-2023-076649. Accessed 7 Mar 2025

Sippy R, Efstathopoulou L, Simes E, Davis M, Howell S, Morris B, Owrid O, Stoll N, Fonagy P, Moore A (2025) Effect of a needs-based model of care on the characteristics of healthcare services in England: the i-THRIVE National Implementation Programme, Epidemiol Psychiatr Sci 34:e21

Steptoe A, Deaton A, Stone AA (2015) Subjective wellbeing, health, and ageing. The Lancet 385(9968):640–648

Swift HJ, Abrams D, Lamont RA, Drury L (2017) The risks of ageism model: How ageism and negative attitudes toward age can be a barrier to active Ageing. Soc Issues Policy Rev 11(1):195–231

The Health Foundation (2025) Mental health trends among working-age people. Available at: https://www.health.org.uk/reports-and-analysis/analysis/mental-health-trends-among-working-age-people. Accessed 18 Feb 2025

The Health Foundation (2026) Why are a growing number of young people who are NEET reporting work-limiting health conditions? Available at: https://www.health.org.uk/reports-and-analysis/analysis/why-are-a-growing-number-of-young-people-who-are-neet-reporting-work. Accessed 11 July 2025

Tong P and An IS (2024) Review of studies applying Bronfenbrenner's bioecological theory in international and intercultural education research, Frontiers in Psychology, 14, Article 1233925. https://doi.org/10.3389/fpsyg.2023.1233925. Accessed 11 Nov 2025.

van Staa A, Peeters M, Sattoe J (2020) On your own feet: a practical framework for improving transitional care and young people's self-management. In: Betz C, Coyne I (eds) Transition from pediatric to adult healthcare services for adolescents and young adults with long-term conditions. Springer, Cham, pp 191–228

Vélez-Agosto NM, Soto-Crespo JG, Vizcarrondo-Oppenheimer M, Vega-Molina S, García Coll C (2017) Bronfenbrenner's bioecological theory revision: Moving culture from the macro into the micro. Perspect Psychol Sci 12(5):900–910

Wolpert M, Harris R, Hodges S, Fuggle P, James R, Wiener A, Munk S (2019) THRIVE Framework for system change. London: CAMHS Press. Accessed 12 Aug 2025.

World Health Organization (WHO) (2023) Mental health of older adults. World Health Organization. Available at: https://www.who.int/news-room/fact-sheets/detail/mental-health-of-older-adults. Accessed 7 Mar 2025

World Health Organization (WHO) (2024) Mental health at work. World Health Organization. Available at: https://www.who.int/news-room/fact-sheets/detail/mental-health-at-work. Accessed 7 Mar 2025

World Health Organization (2025a) Ageing and health. Available at: https://www.who.int/news-room/fact-sheets/detail/ageing-and-health. Accessed 2 Feb 2026

World Health Organization (2025b) Social isolation and loneliness. Available at: https://www.who.int/teams/social-determinants-of-health/demographic-change-and-healthy-ageing/social-isolation-and-loneliness. Accessed 16 Feb 2026

Self-Harm, Suicide and Risk

What Is Self-Harm?

The definition of self-harm refers to the 'intentional act of self-poisoning or self-injury, irrespective of the motivation or apparent purpose of the act and is an expression of emotional distress' (NICE 2025).

Self-harm can be broken into two separate categories, and can be seen explored further within in Table 1 (Clarke et al. 2019):

The total number of self-harm episodes worldwide is unknown (Knipe et al. 2022). In the Adult Psychiatric Morbidity Survey (Morris et al., 2025) the lifetime of self-harm was reported by 10.3% of 16- to 74-year-olds (increasing from 3.4% in 2000). This increase was apparent in both male and female groups. Among people who had self-harmed, cutting was the most reported method.

The prevalence of self-harm was highest in young women, with about 1 in 5 reporting this face to face and one in four reporting by self-completion in 2014. When individuals start to self-harm when young, they are more likely to go on and adopt the behaviour as a long-term strategy for coping (McManus et al. 2019).

Figure 1 demonstrates some of the risk factors for self-harm (NICE 2025).

People who self-injure may take longer to perceive something as painful. People who self-injure may often be able to tolerate painful stimuli for longer periods of time. If you were to ask someone who self-harms, they would likely tell you that their self-injurious behaviours are painful. In this group, however, once the painful stimuli reduce or are removed, they do not return to the same affective state as before. They report a more positive emotional experience—an experience called pain-offset relief (Franklin et al. 2013).

NSSI is a relatively common development amongst young adolescents, and it varies in severity, frequency and associated psychiatric vulnerability (Brañas et al. 2022). Many people who manage their distress by self-harm do not have suicidal intent (Royal College of Psychiatrists 2019). However, there is a direct correlation

R. Bage, *Mental Health Skills for Adult Nurses & Non-Specialist Healthcare Workers*, https://doi.org/10.1007/978-3-032-32835-9_6

Table 1 Self-harm categories

Non-suicidal self-injury	NSSI	Self-injurious behaviours which are performed deliberately, but with no intent to die. Common methods of NSSI can include: Scratching the skin Cutting Burning Head banging Hitting
Self-harm	SH	This is a broader category that includes all intentional self-injury, with or without intent to die.

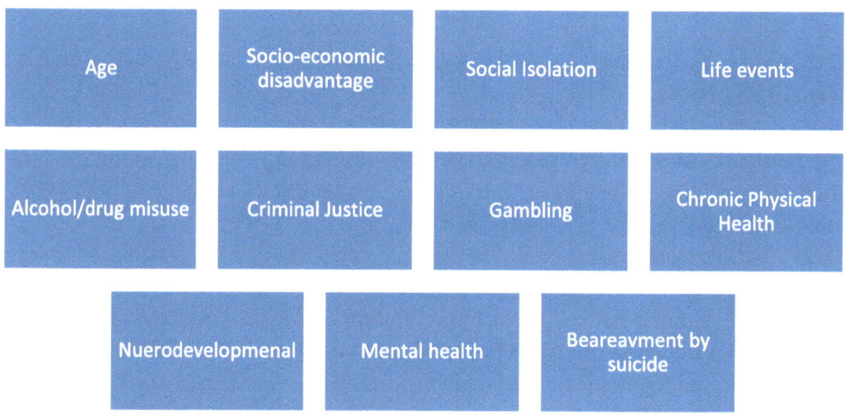
Age
Socio-economic disadvantage
Social Isolation
Life events
Alcohol/drug misuse
Criminal Justice
Gambling
Chronic Physical Health
Nuerodevelopmenal
Mental health
Beareavment by suicide

Fig. 1 Risk factors for self-harm

between deliberate self-harm and suicide attempts (Carroll et al. 2014; Duarte et al. 2019; Hawton et al. 2020). NSSI is one of the most frequent reasons for emergency hospital admission and a strong risk factor for subsequent suicide (Carroll et al. 2014; Hawton et al. 2020).

The National Institute for Health and Care Excellence (NICE) updated guidance for self-harm within the publication of the new NG225 guideline. This new guidance highlights that all people who have self-harmed should receive a psychosocial assessment from a trained mental health professional to identify current needs, strengths of the person and the details of the self-harm event. Mental health professionals are advised not to use risk assessment tools and scales to simply band people into low, medium or high risk for future self-harm or suicide. Instead, mental health professionals should focus on circumstances, strengths and needs to develop a risk formulation (Mughal et al. 2023). Service users who present in acute services should be referred to the most appropriate mental health service for this assessment, e.g., mental health liaison services.

Many people who engage in self-harm do not seek help. This is potentially due to concern about stigmatising attitudes to their self-harm (Lloyd et al. 2018). A 2025 study looking into self-harm stigma in university students identified four main themes: shamed into silence; unspoken but sensed stigma; anticipation and avoidance of stigma; and enduring shadow of stigma (Lewis et al. 2025).

A rapid evidence review of practitioner perspectives to self-harm was completed by the Scottish Government in 2025. Findings from the evidence review and practitioner survey highlighted barriers to accessing supports for individuals who self-harm including fear of self-judgement and self-stigma, and service level issues such as eligibility criteria and long waiting lists (Scottish Government 2025). A 2012 systematic review looking into self-harm and stigma found that attitudes of general hospital staff towards service users who present with self-harm are often negative, mirroring the experiences of service users (Saunders et al. 2012).

Stigma from Caring Professionals

A UK study looking at the perceptions of clinical services in three self-harm online communities found four key themes: access to appropriate services during an episode of self-harm, service preference, fears surrounding disclosure and support (2018). Equally individual responses were highly related to underlying influences of perceived stigma of those who self-injure as well as the external stigma observed within clinical services and the wider public (Williams et al. 2018).

A study found that those who present to A&E after a period of self-harm found four different themes: a failure of the wider system, self-harm raised difficult feelings for staff and service users, human connection and fear of blame (O'Keeffe et al. 2021).

A failure of the wider system—this looks at service users being able to get the specialist care that they need, and staff reported a lack of services to refer service users to. Service users also lacked support in the community to prevent them reaching crisis points (O'Keeffe et al. 2021).

Self-harm raised difficult feelings—self harm often raises difficult feelings for staff and service users in A&E. People often identified that they felt shame when accessing support in A&E settings and staff said they felt powerless. With this, staff attitudes could harden which could be caused by frustration of not being able to help. Some people reported feeling judged or feelings of disapproval (O'Keeffe et al. 2021).

A human connection—people talked about the importance of a human connection, who said that being listened to and having experiences validated was helpful within the A&E department. However, it was noted that some staff felt that this was not their role (O'Keeffe et al. 2021).

Fear of blame—staff reported that there is a fear of risk if somebody takes their own life. Brief question-and-answer risk assessments made staff feel safer and more secure (O'Keeffe et al. 2021).

Working with Somebody Who Has Self-Harmed

Feeling confident in working with people who have self-harmed is important across all branches and professions of healthcare. Self-harm is so common that it is unlikely that any of us will avoid it across our working career. With this in mind, you may want to follow the acronym 'LORES' which is explored further in Fig. 2.

Listen

Ensure that you are listening and engaging with the service user and their family or carers. When people are feeling vulnerable, for whatever reason, human connection is something we will likely all try and seek. By actively engaging in conversation, you will support somebody who is feeling unsafe and vulnerable and offer them help, reassurance and guidance.

Observe

This service user group has higher levels of risk, and as discussed above, self-harm is linked with suicide attempts. It is important to ensure this group is safe in your ward or community environment. Whilst, in most cases, 1:1 observation is not needed, it is important to ensure people are kept safe.

It is also important that these service users are getting the physical health observations they may need. It might be easy to diagnostically overshadow in these cases, but if they are presenting with observations which are not the norm, more investigation is needed.

Refer

It is important to refer on to the relevant mental health services if this is clinically indicated. In most cases, this will likely be the Mental Health Liaison Services within the department. Please always remember that there is a link between self-harm and suicide, and early access to support is always the best plan.

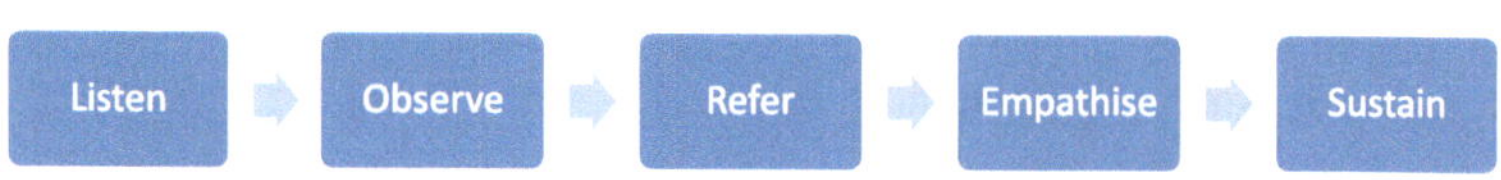

Fig. 2 LORES acronym

Empathise

It is important to remember that people will self-harm for a multitude of different reasons, but it will always be a strategy to process difficult or challenging feelings for people. It is important that people do attend healthcare services when they have self-harmed, and empathising with their situations and needs is an important step to ensure this happens.

Sustain

It is important for any healthcare practitioner to be able to sustain themselves and their work. It is not good for any staff member, service user, or carer to have professionals pushed into compassionate fatigue. It is important to seek support to talk through the more challenging cases, take time to reflect and work as a team to ensure staff are mentally and physically looked after.

Suicide

Suicide in the UK

Between 2012 and 2022, the National Confidential Inquiry into Suicide and Safety in Mental Health (NCISH) was notified of almost 71,000 deaths by suicide or 'undetermined' deaths. Table 2 gives more detail into deaths across the United Kingdom (National Confidential Inquiry into Suicide and Safety in Mental Health 2026).

Suicide in the General Population

There is some variation in the peak age across the UK; however, the highest suicide rates were consistently in the middle-aged groups, especially those between 40 and 49 years old.

Table 2 Suicides in the UK

Country	Deaths by suicide	Deaths by suicide who were currently service users
England	55,705	14,464 (26%)
Scotland	8343	2510 (30%)
Wales	4008	916 (23%)
Northern Ireland	2424	735 (30%)
Jersey	220	45 (41%)

Suicide in Patient Groups

Some of the key social and clinical characteristics are included in Fig. 3 (NCISH 2026):

In total, there were 18,670 people who died by suicide who could be classed as a service user. These are people who have had contact with mental health services within a year of their death. The most common methods of suicide by service users were hanging/strangulation, self-poisoning (most commonly opiates) and jumping/traumatic injuries (National Confidential Inquiry into Suicide and Safety in Mental Health 2026).

The majority of this group were male (65%) and unmarried. Nearly half of those in this group lived alone, and 47% were unemployed. 14% were 65 and over, and 9% were under 25. 5% of this group were migrants, both those seeking permission to stay in the UK or those resident for less than 5 years (National Confidential Inquiry into Suicide and Safety in Mental Health 2026).

There are also some key statistics regarding recent stressors. 17% of people within this category had experienced serious financial problems, and 8% of people had suicide-related internet use. Over half of this group had a comorbid (additional) mental health diagnosis, and there were significant rates of previous alcohol/drug misuse within this group. 62% had a lifetime history of self-harm, 24% of those had been seen by the emergency department for self-harm (National Confidential Inquiry into Suicide and Safety in Mental Health 2026).

The primary diagnosis of mental health service users who died by suicide varies. The largest group (39%) is those who had a diagnosis of an affective disorder, either a depressive illness or bipolar disorder. Schizophrenia diagnosis made up 15% of this group, and personality disorder 11% (National Confidential Inquiry into Suicide and Safety in Mental Health 2026).

Nearly half of this group (46%) had been in contact with services in the week before their death. In the majority of service users, their immediate risk of suicide was classified as not present or low in their final service contact. In the 2012–2022 period, 27% of service users who died by suicide did so in acute care settings (in-patients, crisis resolution/home treatment, recently discharged from in-patient care).

There were 1004 in-patient deaths by suicide, representing 5% of patient suicides overall. 40% of these service users died whilst on the ward, 50% died after having left the ward with staff agreement, and 10% of these had left the ward without staff agreement or left with agreement but did not return. 34% of this group had been detained under the Mental Health Act. 90% of these deaths were by hanging/strangulation/asphyxia (National Confidential Inquiry into Suicide and Safety in Mental Health 2026).

Fig. 3 Suicide risk factors

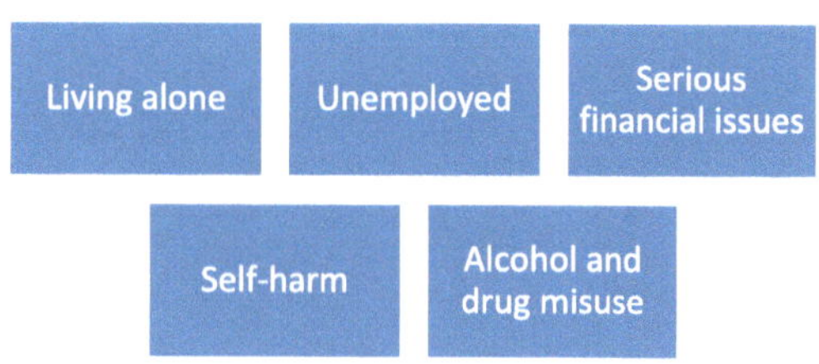
Living alone
Unemployed
Serious financial issues
Self-harm
Alcohol and drug misuse

2317 service users across 2012–2022 died within 3 months of discharge from mental health services (National Confidential Inquiry into Suicide and Safety in Mental Health 2026).

Bereaved Service Users

In 2012–2022, there were 1312 mental health service users who died by suicide and had been recently bereaved (within the last 3 months). This group were more often female service users, with a higher median age (49 years). There was a higher proportion in this category who were widowed and living alone. The most common diagnosis within this group was a depressive illness, but many also had a diagnosis of adjustment disorder. A history of alcohol misuse was common. The majority of this group had been prescribed antidepressants, and 20% were receiving psychological therapy. This group were more likely to die of self-poisoning compared to other service users and were more likely to die on or near the family member/friend's death anniversary. 26% of this group had missed their last appointment with services (National Confidential Inquiry into Suicide and Safety in Mental Health 2026).

Suicide Worldwide

The World Health Organization (2021) estimates that 720,000 globally die by suicide each year. Suicide is the third leading cause of death amongst young people aged between 15–29 years. More than 50% of global suicides happened before the age of 50 years (World Health Organization 2025).

Approximately three quarters of global suicides occurred in low- and middle-income countries in 2021. Experiencing conflict, disaster, violence, abuse, loss, or isolation is strongly associated with suicidal behaviours. Suicide rates are also high among vulnerable groups who have experienced discrimination, e.g., refugees, migrants, indigenous peoples, LGBT communities, intersex persons and prisoners.

Attempting suicide is a punishable offence in many countries across sub-Saharan Africa, the Middle East and southeast Asia. This can lead to the underreporting of deaths by suicide. (Mishara and Weisstub 2016).

Risk Assessment

Harm minimisation is central to the risk assessment process and any subsequent risk management plans. This assessment should contain the common themes such as self-harm, self-neglect, suicide and violence to self and others. A risk assessment should be completed collaboratively with the service users and carers (Moone and Trenoweth 2024).

Case Study

Amelia is a 28-year-old woman who presents to the Emergency Department following self-inflicted injury to her wrist. This is her fifth attendance in recent weeks, with four previous presentations involving similar behaviour. Each visit has occurred during periods of heightened emotional distress, often late in the evening, and typically following interpersonal conflict or feelings of being overwhelmed. Although the physical injuries have been minor, her repeated attendance has raised significant concern regarding her emotional wellbeing and her ability to remain safe in the community.

Amelia has a diagnosis of a personality disorder and is currently under the care of the local Community Mental Health Team. Despite this, engagement has been inconsistent. She frequently misses scheduled appointments, explaining that she finds structured contact difficult and prefers to seek help during moments of crisis. This pattern has resulted in a reliance on emergency services rather than planned therapeutic support, limiting opportunities for sustained intervention.

Her social support network is limited. Amelia lives alone in a small, rented flat and recent tension with her family has reduced the informal support she previously relied on. She reports feeling isolated and describes her home environment as a source of anxiety rather than stability. Housing insecurity is emerging as a concern, as she has fallen behind on rent during periods of poor mental health.

What are the current risks with Amelia?
What questions would you want to ask Amelia?
Would you want to refer Amelia to mental health services?

Risk in mental health is often thought of through four different lenses, as seen in Fig. 4.

Risk to Self/Others

In this, we consider some of the risks that might be seen as 'risk to self'. This includes things such as self-neglect (e.g. not eating or drinking), self-harm, suicide and substance misuse.

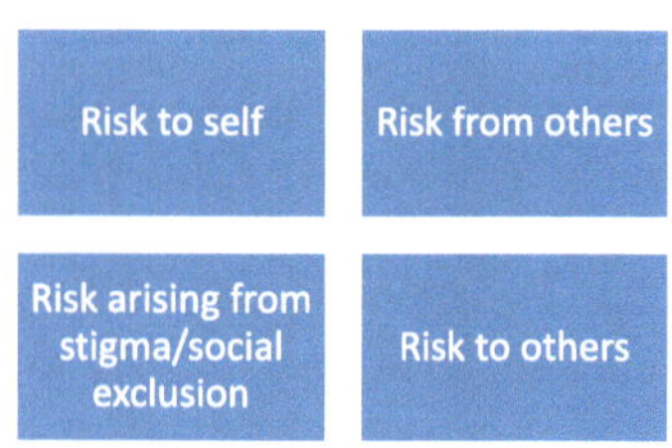
Risk to self
Risk from others
Risk arising from stigma/social exclusion
Risk to others

Fig. 4 Four different lenses in mental health care

Risk to Others

We also consider risk to others such as aggression, violence (e.g. domestic violence), neglect of dependents and exploiting others (e.g. catfishing).

Risk from Others

This can be things such as physical violence, psychological or sexual abuse, intimate partner violence, victimisation, exploitation.

Risk Arising from Stigma/Social Exclusion

This can be things such as losing contact with friends and family, or children. This can also include things such as loss of employment or isolation.

Risk Associated with Health and Care

This can be things such as poor physical health, disengagement, non-compliance and the adverse effects of medication and treatment.

The advised approach for mental health assessment by mental health professionals is structured professional judgement (DH 2007). A structured professional combines the evidence (e.g., risk factors) with an individualised assessment which looks at circumstances, needs and strengths. Some practitioners may wish to use this alongside structured assessment tools (Butler and Haslam 2024). Risk assessment tools, categories and scales cannot accurately identify those at further risk of self-harm or self-harm and should not be used to determine future management or treatment.

Mental health assessments are normally completed by mental health nurses or practitioners. However, NMC Future Nurse (2018) identifies that at the point of qualifying, adult student nurses should have the field level knowledge of the following skills in mental health:

Part 1: Procedures for assessing people's needs for person-centred care

1. *Use evidence-based, best practice approaches to take a history, observe, recognise and accurately assess people of all ages:*
   1.1 *mental health and wellbeing status*
      1.1.1 *signs of mental and emotional distress or vulnerability*
      1.1.2 *cognitive health status and wellbeing*
      1.1.3 *signs of cognitive distress and impairment*
      1.1.4 *behavioural distress-based needs*
      1.1.5 *signs of mental and emotional distress including agitation, aggression and challenging behaviour*
      1.1.6 *signs of self-harm and/or suicidal ideation*

Future Nurse (NMC 2018) has been criticised for being incredibly specific in parts, and vague in language and requirements in others (Warrender 2024). It is not clear what NMC Future Nurse means by 'field-level knowledge' of being able to do the competencies listed above. However, it is clear that at times, adult nurses do complete mental health risk assessment.

There are some aides-memoire however, that can be helpful in supporting your interpersonal, interviewing and observational skills in gathering information from services users, carers and professional sources. HI-RISK offers a good aide-memoire (Butler and Haslam 2024).

History of Risk Behaviour

You will want to take the opportunity to explore the history of their behaviours, and what has brought them in. For example, if they have attended with self-harm, you may want to explore what they did and have they done this before? (Butler and Haslam 2024).

Intent

You will want to explore the intent behind the behaviour. As previously discussed, some deliberate self-harm is done where there is no suicidal intent, and some where they have done this in an attempt to end their own life (Butler and Haslam 2024).

Recency and Frequency

You will want to clarify at this point whether this has happened before. If it has happened before, it is important to clarify how often it is happening and how recently they have done this before (Butler and Haslam 2024).

Ideation

You will want to investigate the ideation further behind the deliberate self-harm. Have they been thinking about suicide or thinking about escaping (Butler and Haslam 2024).

Severity/Impact

You will want to explore the severity of the injury, and if this has been a more severe injury than previously. You will want to explore whether they were in control of their actions, or whether the result of the injury is more severe than they have intended (Butler and Haslam 2024).

Knowledge of the Person

This is when you will want to explore your knowledge of the person, or other's knowledge of the person. You may want to look whether they have presented previously in your service with similar injuries or intent. You will also want to understand if there have been similar circumstances, triggers or planning/understanding of their behaviour.

Formulation is a key feature in risk management and is the process that mental health nurses go through to document risk and formulate a plan. Working together, a formulation gives the opportunity to consider safety and risk concerns, and protective factors in relation to an individual. This helps to support clinicians to make a better judgement about their situation and behaviours and formulate a shared evidence-based care and safety plan.

Formulation considers five different interweaving sections:

Presenting Issues

This is the background of what brought your patient to the department. This will include factors such as their symptoms and their impact/treatment.

Predisposing Factors (Vulnerability and Historical Factors)

This is the factors that are contributing to the person's risk. This might include things such as family history (e.g., dad ended life by suicide), trauma, brain injury, or personal beliefs. This will include both static and stable risk factors.

Precipitating Factors (Trigger Factors)

This will include trigger factors to today's presenting issue. This might be something like stressful work situation, relationship break up, or financial difficulties. This might also include things such as alcohol or drug misuse. This will include both static and stable risk factors.

Perpetuating Factors (Maintaining Factors)

This will be the factors that maintain the current difficulties. This could be behavioural patterns, insomnia, ongoing drug or alcohol misuse, or cognitive patterns. This will include both static and stable risk factors.

Positive/Protective Factors

This will include a service user's strengths or supports that may help to mitigate some of the factors of the illness or difficulties. This could be personal strengths or characteristics, hobbies, or social supports (Butler and Haslam 2024).

Positive Risk Taking

Taking risks is a fundamental part of how humans function. Therapeutic risk-taking enables service users to make decisions about their own level of safety and ability to pursue different goals (Felton et al. 2017).

The principles of therapeutic risk-taking are as follows:

1. Decision-making is joint between professionals and service users.
2. Information is shared clearly to promote informed choice.
3. Service users' capabilities and strengths are drawn on.
4. The outcomes of a decision are managed by effective assessment and collaborative planning.
5. It is accepted that risk-taking may result in positive achievements, not just negative events (Felton et al. 2017).

The assessment and management of risks with service-users is one of the important elements of modern psychiatric practice. Equally, it may be the aspect the public and the media have the most concern with. However, conceptualisation of risk remains dominated by whether the service-user is a danger to themselves or others (Felton et al. 2017). This leaves professionals often acting as a mechanism of control, identifying, quantifying and containing risk. This aspect often leaves service-users not visible, or ignored, in the decision-making processes about risk (Felton et al. 2017).

It should not be underestimated the shift that it takes to promote therapeutic risk-taking in clinical practice. This is not only in mental health practice, but any positive risks that you might make in your own practice (Felton et al. 2017).

Reflective Questions

Do you make any positive risks within your own clinical practice?

What sways whether you make clinical risks in your own practice?

The shift in positive risk taking in mental health practice requires practitioners to shift their thinking in regard to mental illness, role of the practitioner and the individual service user. These decisions are often made with different legal, organisational and professional constraints, and considering safety, restriction and opportunity. Positive risk taking is often where there are huge dilemmas in mental health practice (Felton et al. 2017).

Examples of where positive risk taking may be used:

1. Discharge of a service user—there may be some very real concerns about the discharge of a service user, and concerns about dangers in the community (e.g., drug or alcohol misuse), however these risks will be considered on an individual basis.
2. There may be a discussion about a service user managing their own medication in the community. A service user may ask to change from depot injection to oral medication, and there are significant concerns related to this. This would be considered a positive risk.
3. You may have a conversation in practice about a service user who has had a significant period of unwellness, including with hospitalisation, about returning to the work or voluntary sector. It is well known that work is a positive influence, but also comes with risk about stress, workload balance and symptom flare-ups. As part of these conversations, you may discuss things such as reasonable adjustments, phased returns and structure.
4. Another positive risk that might be taken in mental health may be around home leave or overnight leave. This may be an appropriate next step for people working towards discharge. However, there may also be triggers or risks with this and boundaries may be discussed with the service user prior to this being started.

There are many barriers to positive risk-taking in mental health practice. There continue to be organisational policies which do not encourage positive risk-taking (Boardman and Roberts 2014). It is important that there is board-level endorsement of positive, recovery-orientated approaches to risk. Equally, we also need to ensure we have good mechanisms to record and monitor decisions that have been made.

The terms 'risk' and 'risk management' can be barriers to considering risk in a collaborative approach. We, as clinicians, need to move away from terminology such as 'What are your risks?' to 'What do you need in place to stay safe?' (Boardman and Roberts 2014).

Work from Correia and Jackson (2021) gives some good questions to consider when conducting a risk assessment:

Have you ever attempted to take your own life or harm yourself in the past?
Do you use alcohol and/or other illicit substances?
Do you have any current mental health-related difficulties?
Do you have any current physical health conditions?
Have you ever known anyone who has taken their own life or self-harmed?
Do you ever feel hopeless and have thoughts of being better off dead?

Do you have any specific plans to harm yourself? Do you have images about completing this?
How likely are you to act on these thoughts at the moment? Can you rate intent on a scale of 0–10?
What has stopped you from acting on these thoughts in the past?

Children and adolescents: as well as asking the above questions, it is important to clarify who else knows about the risk (i.e. peers or trusted adult) and, depending on the answer, discuss limits to confidentiality and devise a safety plan that involves making a trusted adult aware—this depends also on the nature of the risk and individual circumstances. It would also be important to clarify the patient's understanding of the consequences of certain acts e.g., whether they understand it could lead to death.

As part of the questions above, you will want to understand the recency, severity, frequency and persistency of the thoughts.

Safety Planning Interventions

Safety planning is a structured and proactive way to help people plan a range of activities and sources they can use at the right time to help prevent crises.

Stanley et al. (2008) advise that safety plans should involve the following factors:

1. Recognising warning signs that might be present prior to an impending crisis.
2. Identifying and using internal coping strategies.
3. Using contact with people to help to distract (without discussion of self-harm/suicide).
4. Discuss with friends/family when crisis and suicidality can be discussed.
5. Mental health professional contact details.
6. Ensuring the environment is safer or avoiding more risk environments.

The most recent NICE guideline in relation to self-harm (NG225) also discusses the importance of having a written, prioritised list of coping strategies or sources of support (National Institute for Health and Care Excellence 2022). This is a list that people who have self-harmed can use to avoid or end a crisis. They discuss that elements within this safety plan should include:

- Recognising warning signs.
- Listing coping strategies.
- Friends and family members.
- Contacting mental health services.
- Limiting access to self-harm methods.

Sensory boxes or 'self-soothe' boxes can play part of a successful safety planning. Self-help toolkits include sensory objects, distractions and prompts to help them manage the urge to self-harm. Creative prompts can also prove to be successful—colouring books, pencils, or personal items that may help trigger or distract to more positive memories (Fenton et al. 2024).

Prompt

You have been tasked with producing a self-soothe box for yourself. Think of some items that you may want to put in this box. You might find some of the prompts helpful below:

- Photos of people/pets/happy memories.
- A piece of personal writing about happy memories or occasions.
- A letter from yourself.
- Notes or card from people that you care about.
- Positive quotes, affirmations, song lyrics.
- Glitter jar.
- Colouring activities.
- Sensory toys (NHS Best for You 2026; Fenton et al. 2024).

Documentation and Legal

Mental Health Act

The Mental Health Act (MHA) provides the legal basis for detaining and treating individuals with mental disorders without their consent when necessary for their health, safety, or the protection of others.

The Mental Health Act was revised from the Mental Health Act 1983 to the Mental Health Act 2025. This was after the independent review of the Mental Health Act was published in 2018. The review drivers were to reduce detention rates and the inequality within some ethnic minority groups in the use of the MHA. Implementation of the new Act will take place over the next 10 years. The Mental Health Act is the current legislation for England and Wales only (Cronin et al. 2017).

Summary of some of the key elements of the Mental Health Act

Section 2

- A patient may be admitted to hospital and detained there if he/she is suffering from a mental disorder of a nature or degree that warrants a period of assessment for a limited period.
- He/she needs to be detained in the interests of his/her own health or safety or with a view to the protection of other persons.

- Detention is agreed by AMHP and two approved mental health doctors.
- This will be for a period not exceeding 28 days (*Mental Health Act* 1983 (*as amended by the Mental Health Act* 2007)).

Section 3

- A patient may be admitted to hospital and detained there if he/she is suffering from a mental disorder of a nature or degree that it is appropriate to receive medication treatment in a hospital.
- He/she needs to be detained in the interests of his/her own health or safety or with a view to protection of other persons.
- Detention is agreed by AMHP and two approved mental health psychiatrists.
- This will be for a period not exceeding 6 months, although unlike section 2, this can be extended (*Mental Health Act* 1983 (*as amended by the Mental Health Act* 2007)).

Section 4

- A patient can be detained in an emergency by an emergency application by an approved mental health professional or by the nearest relative of the patient.
- This is for a period of no more than 72 hours from when the person is admitted to hospital (*Mental Health Act* 1983 (*as amended by the Mental Health Act* 2007)).

Nurses' Holding Power (Section 5(4))

This is commonly referred to as the 'nurses holding power'. 5(4) is only able to be used by nurses registered in either Sub-Part 1 or 2 of the register maintained under article 5 of the Nursing and midwifery Order 2001—this means any nurse under sub-part mental health or learning disabilities nursing. This is for a period of up to 6 hours to arrange an assessment (*Mental Health Act* 1983 (*as amended by the Mental Health Act* 2007)).

One of the challenges with the nurses holding power (Section 5(4)) is that this is not usable by adult nurses. As more adult nurses choose to transition into mental health settings, this becomes a challenge to manage.

Doctors' Holding Power (Section 5(2))

This is commonly referred to as the 'doctors holding power'. This allows responsible doctor or approved the ability to detain someone in hospital for up to 72 hours for the purpose of making arrangements for assessment for detention under either section 2 or 3 of the MHA. Holding powers can only be used with service users who have already been admitted to a hospital and cannot be used with outpatients (*Mental Health Act* 1983 (*as amended by the Mental Health Act* 2007)).

Section 135

Section 135 is when police are able to enter a person's home and take you to a place of safety for a mental health assessment. This is only able to take place when a warrant is in place from the magistrate's court. The police can keep you at the place of safety for up to 24 hours, which can be extended for a further 12 hours if there is difficulty arranging the assessment (*Mental Health Act* 1983 (*as amended by the Mental Health Act* 2007)).

Section 136

Section 136 allows the police to take up to keep you at a place of safety. They can do this without a warrant if they believe you have a mental disorder, you are in a public place and you are in need of immediate care or control. If possible, police should have discussed with a nurse, doctor or other clinician before detaining. The police can keep you at the place of safety for up to 24 hours, which can be extended for a further 12 hours if there is difficulty arranging the assessment (*Mental Health Act* 1983 (*as amended by the Mental Health Act* 2007)).

Independent Mental Health Advocate (IMHA)

An IMHA is an independent advocate who is trained in the Mental Health Act and supports people to understand their rights under the Act. It helps service users to participate in decision-making, especially around their care and treatment. The advocates are not employed by the NHS or healthcare provider, and the advice they provide is free (PohWER 2022). You can receive support from an IMHA if:

- You are detained under the Mental Health Act, excluding the short terms sections—4, 5(2), 5(4), 135 or 136.
- A conditionally discharged restricted service user.
- Subject to Guardianship under the Act.
- Receiving Supervised Community Treatment.
- Being considered for treatment to which a section 57 applies.
- Under 18 and being considered for either electro-convulsive treatment or any other treatment to which section 58A applies.

People may benefit from an IMHA to:

- Understand their section further, and understand how to appear against it under the Mental Health Review Tribunal process.
- To understand their rights and the safeguards that apply.
- To understand the medical treatment you are receiving or treatment that might be given.
- To understand requirements that would apply in connection with the treatment (PohWER 2022).

Did You Know?

There is lots of diversity in the mental health legislation different countries use. For example, in the Republic of Ireland and Ontario, only one medical recommendation is needed for detention. England and Wales detention period for assessment is also one of the longest, with Republic of Ireland and Ontario being much shorter at just 7 days (Cronin et al. 2017).

Common Questions About the Mental Health Act

Can 5(2) or 5(4) be used when a service user is in Accident and Emergency?

No. A + E classifies as an outpatient department, and they have not been admitted to the hospital. You cannot use 5(2) or 5(4) in this environment.

Can you use 5(4) when there is an approved doctor in the building?

No. This is for use when the arrival time of the doctor is likely to be after the patient leaves and it is not possible to persuade the patient to stay any longer.

What is a 'Place of Safety'?

This can be places such as a hospital, care home, your own house or any other suitable premises if the manager agrees. Police stations can still be used but only when there is an imminent risk of injury to yourself or others. If a person has been taken to the police station, their wellbeing must be checked every 30 minutes, and a review must be done hourly on the suitability of the police station. Police stations must never be used for under 18s (*Mental Health Act* 1983 (*as amended by the Mental Health Act* 2007)).

Mental Capacity Act

The MCA came into force in 2007 and has been designed to protect and restore power to vulnerable people who lack the capacity to make certain decisions (SCIE 2026). It provides a comprehensive framework for decision-making of over 16s. The Act applies in England and Wales only and applies to all decisions taken on behalf of somebody who permanently or temporarily lacks capacity to make decisions themselves (NHS Health Research Authority 2026).

The main principles of the Mental Capacity Act are as follows:

- A person must be assumed to have capacity unless it is established that he lacks capacity.
- A person is not to be treated as unable to make a decision unless all practicable steps to help him/her to do so have been taken without success.
- A person is not to be treated as unable to make a decision merely because he or she makes an unwise decision.
- An act done, or decision made, under this Act for or on behalf of a person who lacks capacity must be done, or made, in his/her best interests.
- Before the act is done, or the decision is made, regard must be had to whether the purpose for which it is needed can be effectively achieved in a way that is less restrictive of the person's rights and freedom of action (MCA, 2005).

The two-stage functional test of capacity is a supported approach of undertaking an assessment of capacity.

1. Is the person able to make the decision (with support if required)?
2. If they cannot, is there an impairment or disturbance in the functioning of their mind or brain? Is the person's inability to make the decision because of the impairment or disturbance?

Table 3 Implementation of the Mental Capacity Act

Issue	Examples
Busy clinical environments	You may experience pressures within environments to make quick clinical decisions which may lead you to feel pressured to make shortcuts in capacity assessments
Insufficient training	Whilst you may have had training in capacity assessments, if you are not using regularly, you may need further training or an update
Misconceptions	There may be misconception that certain conditions may imply lack of capacity or that you cannot have capacity if you have a certain condition or illness
Autonomy vs. protection	You may feel ethical dilemmas in balancing autonomy or patient choice and a need for protection
Litigation	Some cases may make you feel as if you are at risk of a legal case or further repercussions.
Communication	You may feel underconfident or unskilled in understanding the different ways people may communicate their decisions. There may also be cases where you need to use interpreters or sign language interpreters which you may struggle to access
Inclusion/ exclusion	Some family members may be excluded from the decision-making or insufficiently involved in the decision-making
Disagreements	There may be differing views within your team, between teams or within family groups
Inadequate record keeping	There may be inconsistencies within the documentation of capacity assessments and best interest assessments
Lack of specialist support	There may be limited access to specialist advice, or you may feel unable to contact the professionals you need to help support the process
Lack of guidelines	There may be unclear or inadequate policies or procedures within your workplace which make it difficult to conduct the MCA

The person should be classified as unable to make the relevant decision if they are unable to:

Understand the information that is given to them.
Retain that information long enough to be able to make the decision.
Weight up the information available to be able to make the decision.
Communicate their decision—this could be talking, sign language or blinking (SCIE 2022).

NHS England (2026) documented a number of barriers to effective implementation of the MCA in acute care which will be discussed in the Table 3 (NHS England 2026):

The Interaction of MHA and MCA

There are some key differences between the Mental Capacity Act (2005) and the Mental Health Act 1983/2025, which are noted within Table 4 (Wheeler 2018).

The interaction between the Mental Health Act 1983 (and subsequently the Mental Health Act 2025) and the Mental Capacity Act 2005 can cause challenging and complex issues. The MHA is often viewed as a very coercive 'compulsory power' and the MCA as a substitute decision-making law that is 'empowering' (Series 2025).

Norfolk and Suffolk NHS Foundation Trust Versus HJ (2023)

HJ had long-standing mental health problems (bipolar) and various physical health problems. HJ's mental health was categorised by psychotic symptoms, delusions, hallucinations and very challenging behaviours. HJ had medication administered covertly under section 4 of the MCA or via depot injection (at times under restraint). This case was brought to court to determine whether it was lawful to deprive HJ of her liberty while healthcare professionals administered enemas for constipation. This case focussed specifically on the overlap between the MHA and MCA on physical healthcare. HJ was detained under section 3 of the MHA (Curtice 2025).

Table 4 Interaction between MHA and MCA

	Mental Health Act	Mental Capacity Act
Age	The Mental Health is applicable for citizens of any age	The Mental Capacity Act applies to citizens over the age of 16 (although some elements are only relevant to those over the age of 18)
Threshold	Person is currently suffering from a mental disorder defined by the Act.	Triggered by establishing a person lacks capacity to make a particular decision
Clinical application	MHA is linked with psychiatric training and practice Acts in parallel with the MCA on acute hospital wards.	In theory, provides authority for the treatment of any physical or mental disorder in a patient who lacks capacity, but when compulsion is needed to provide treatment for mental disorder the MHA becomes a preferable authority
Best interests	The MHA 1983 does not employ the phrase 'best interest'	The principle of acting in a patient's best interests lies at the core the MCA
Parental responsibility	MHA has rules about parental responsibility for children—and advises not to rely on parental consent that overrides the refusal of a competent young person who lack capacity	The MCA ensures decisions are made on the best interest of a service user. For under 18s, parental responsibility will usually be sufficient to allow them to consent or refuse treatment on their behalf, but when this is not possible, the MCA may be used

HJ's constipation was not a direct consequence of her mental health, but instead various physical health conditions. Usual treatment would have involved diet, exercise, laxatives and enemas as needed, as well as avoidance of any medications that may cause constipation. In HJ's case, a plan was made to increase laxatives to try and avoid the use of enemas which often had to be given under restraint (requiring five members of staff). However, increased laxatives caused peristaltic contractions and discomfort and had to be reduced (Curtice 2025).

The judge in this case concurred with the trust's position that HJ's constipation was not caused by her mental ill health, and there was no documented change in her mental health once she had received the enema. It was agreed that the administration of enemas fell outside of the scope of section 63 of the MHA (Treatment not requiring consent). However, the judgement was satisfied that the MCA provided a sufficient framework for the lawful actions of the trust and staff. The Judge made a declaration under section 15 of the MCA (Power to make declarations) that the trust was acting lawfully in administering enemas to HJ in accordance with relevant treatment plans (Curtice 2025).

Manchester University Hospitals NHS Foundation Trust Versus JS and Others

JS was a teenager with complex mental health issues and considered a risk to herself and was thus receiving treatment at a specialist child and adolescent psychiatric unit. JS was detained shortly after discharge on two occasions under s.136 due to self-harm and suicide. JS was then detained under s.2 to an adult medical ward to treat her physical health following an overdose. JS remained on this ward for a number of weeks, well past the expiry of the s.2. On this ward, there were several more self-harm attempts, and she was started on antipsychotic, antidepressants, and a care plan of 'restrictions'. The Trust made an application to the Court of Protection for an order under 2.16 of the MCA, in order for her to stay in hospital and under the restrictions of the care plan (RCPLegal 2023).

The Court found that JS had been unlawfully deprived of her liberty after the s.2 MHA authority had expired. JS was found to have limited mental capacity and the care provision in hospital was most suitable option for JS at the time. JS was within the scope of the MHA and should have been treated under this act and was ineligible for detention under the MCA (RCPLegal 2023).

Sherwood Forest Hospitals NHS Foundation Trust & Nottingham University Hospitals NHS Trust Versus H (2020)

This case was based on a woman with bipolar disorder and advanced skin cancer, which required surgery. The court found that she did lack capacity to consent to the surgery, but it was in her best interests. In this case, there was a significant delay in taking this case to Court as clinicians were perplexed as to in which circumstances Mrs. H could be forced or coerced into attending for treatment.

Key Points

Under section 63 of the MHA (treatment not requiring consent), treatment for physical disorders can occur without consent where there is a clear causal connection in that the physical disorder is a symptom or manifestation of the mental illness (Curtice 2025).

For service users who are detained and the physical disorder is not the primary or subsidiary cause of a mental disorder (totally unrelated), section 63 cannot be used (Curtice 2025).

For a detained service user under the MHA and where section 63 does not apply for physical health treatment, and they are unable to consent, then the MCA framework will apply (Curtice 2025).

Reflective Practice

Working with people who have tried to end their life by suicide, completed deliberate self-injury, or detained/treated under a piece of legislation is challenging. All of these things come with different stressors and will impact us all in different ways. Many of us will have our own experiences or family experiences of poor mental health, and working in such an environment can be triggering. Many of these more challenging cases will stay with us for a long time. I certainly still think of some more emotional cases still, even 10 years on.

It is important to have the opportunity to work about these stressors in our own clinical practice. Mental health nurses will routinely get the opportunity to have clinical supervision within their working environment, which sadly is not always replicated in other environments. There is something extremely beneficial to discuss through challenging cases, things which may have pushed you, or cases that may have caused you increased anxiety or stress.

Scwartz rounds are a newer idea in practice. Schwartz rounds provide a structured forum where staff, whether clinical or not, can come together to discuss the more emotional and social aspects of working in health and social care. They can be helpful in reducing the feelings of stress and isolation which impact on our ability to provide compassionate care to service users. Equally, they can be useful to remind us why we work in healthcare, even in the tough moments (The Point of Care Foundation 2026).

As a lecturer, I encourage my students to reflect on their day. One of the strategies I encourage within my students is to write down at least one good thing and one more challenging thing that happened in their day after their shift. I value this technique at the end of the shift to help give students (and any clinicians) separation at the end of the day.

Key Learning Points

Self-harm is a common occurrence and often happens for complex reasons. You should remember that this is not always a suicide attempt and is often used as a way to handle unmanageable emotions.

Do not rely on risk tools—rely on your own assessment. Talk to service users that you may come across and explore their risks collaboratively and with a good-quality biopsychosocial assessment.

The way practitioners, of any fields or speciality, come across can often be a barrier to people receiving or presenting for care. We must remember that the human connection is the most important element of our practice.

Mental health is often first spotted and identified in non-mental health practice. It is imperative that any practitioners are looking for signs of distress, agitation, self-harm or suicidal thoughts.

Know your boundaries and overlap between Mental Health Act and the Mental Capacity Act.

It is important that we do not become risk-averse. Positive risk-taking is an important part of all practitioners' practice. You may be involved in positive risk-taking decisions such as managing medication, service users' going home, or engaging with other activities of daily life.

Conclusion

Self-harm, suicide and risk assessments are some of the most complex areas in mental health practice. They are often emotionally charged and ethically challenging for any practitioner. This chapter has highlighted the importance of understanding these experiences in the wider context of mental ill health, trauma, social adversity and personal distress. By exploring the functions of self-harm, we can learn how to respond in ways that are compassionate, person-centred and focussed on understanding rather than judgement. Fundamentally, we need to remember how we would want to be treated if we were experiencing intense emotional pain, fear, or hopelessness ourselves. Developing empathy, therapeutic communication and emotional awareness is therefore central to effective practice.

The chapter has also explored the significant role of legal and ethical frameworks, particularly the Mental Health Act and Mental Capacity Act, in guiding practice. Understanding these laws, including their boundaries and interactions, ensures that practitioners act lawfully, respectfully and in the best interests of those they support. Case law examples illustrate the real-world complexities involved in balancing autonomy, protection, dignity and the least restrictive approach. Practitioners must often make difficult decisions in situations where risk can fluctuate rapidly, highlighting the importance of sound professional judgement, collaborative working and ongoing review.

Finally, the emotional impact of working in this field cannot be overstated. Reflective practice, supervision and initiatives such as Schwartz Rounds are vital in sustaining staff wellbeing and enabling compassionate, ethical care. Open discussions around emotional resilience, burnout and moral distress are increasingly important within healthcare environments where practitioners are frequently exposed to trauma and crisis. By integrating clinical knowledge, legal literacy, reflective awareness and relational practice, practitioners are better equipped to navigate uncertainty, respond safely to distress and contribute positively to the lives of those at risk.

References

Boardman J, Roberts G (2014) Risk, safety and recovery. London: Centre for Mental Health and NHS Confederation Mental Health Network. Available at: http://www.cpa.org.uk/information/reviews/CPA-ageism_and_age_discrimination_in_primary_and_community_health_care-report.pdf. Accessed 21 July 2026

Brañas MJAA, Croci MS, Murray GE, Choi-Kain LW (2022) The relationship between self-harm and suicide in adolescents and young adults. Psychiatr Ann 52(8):311–317. https://doi.org/10.3928/00485713-20220715-01. Accessed 7 Mar 2025

Butler J, Haslam M (2024) 'Mental health risk assessment: A personalised approach'. In: Wright, K.M. and McKeown, M. (eds.) Essentials of Mental Health Nursing. 2nd edn. London: SAGE, pp. 499–518

Carroll R, Metcalfe C, Gunnell D (2014) Hospital presenting self-harm and risk of fatal and non-fatal repetition: systematic review and meta-analysis. PLoS One 9(2):e89944. https://doi.org/10.1371/journal.pone.0089944. Accessed 7 Mar 2025

Clarke S, Allerhand LA, Berk MS (2019) Recent advances in understanding and managing self-harm in adolescents. F1000Res 8(1):1794. https://doi.org/10.12688/f1000research.19868.1. Accessed 7 Mar 2025

Correia R, Jackson D (2021) Risk to self: Identifying and managing risk of suicide and self-harm, BJPsych Advances 27(2):126–136. https://doi.org/10.1192/bja.2020.48. Accessed 21 July 2026

Cronin T, Gouda P, McDonald C, Hallahan B (2017) A comparison of mental health legislation in five developed countries: A narrative review. Ir J Psychol Med 34(4):261–269. https://doi.org/10.1017/ipm.2017.48. Accessed 21 July 2026

Curtice M (2025) The interface between the Mental Health Act and Mental Capacity Act: physical health treatment. BJPsych Adv 31(1):53–61. https://doi.org/10.1192/bja.2023.66. Accessed 7 Mar 2025

Department of Health (2007) Best practice in managing risk: principles and guidance for best practice in the assessment and management of risk to self and others in mental health services. Department of Health, London. Accessed 12 Oct 2025

Duarte TA, Paulino S, Almeida C, Gomes HS, Santos N, Gouveia-Pereira M (2019) Self-harm as a predisposition for suicide attempts: a study of adolescents' deliberate self-harm, suicidal ideation, and suicide attempts. Psychiatry Res 287:112553. https://doi.org/10.1016/j.psychres.2019.112553. Accessed 2 Mar 2025

Felton A, Wright N, Stacey G (2017) Therapeutic risk-taking: A justifiable choice, BJPsych Adv 23(2):81–88. https://doi.org/10.1192/apt.bp.115.015701. Accessed 21 July 2026

Fenton C, Holmes J, Taylor A, Jackson Z (2024) A systematic review of the use, acceptability, perceived effectiveness and effectiveness of self-help toolkits. Issues Ment Health Nurs 45(8):868–880. https://doi.org/10.1080/01612840.2024.2377229. Accessed 2 Mar 2025

Franklin JC, Puzia ME, Lee KM, Lee GE, Hanna EK, Spring VL. Prinstein MJ (2013) The Nature of Pain Offset Relief in Nonsuicidal Self-Injury. Clin Psychol Sci 1(2):110–119. https://doi.org/10.1177/2167702612474440. Accessed 21 July 2026

Hawton K, Bale L, Brand F, Townsend E, Ness J, Waters K, Clements C, Kapur N, Geulayov G (2020) Mortality in children and adolescents following presentation to hospital after non-fatal self-harm in the Multicentre Study of Self-harm: a prospective observational cohort study.

Lancet Child Adolesc Health 4(2):111–120. https://doi.org/10.1016/s2352-4642(19)30373-6. Accessed 2 Mar 2025

Health Research Authority (2026) Mental Capacity Act. Available at: https://www.hra.nhs.uk/planning-and-improving-research/policies-standards-legislation/mental-capacity-act/. Accessed 21 July 2026

Knipe D, John A, Padmanathan P, Eyles E, Dekel D, Higgins JPT, Bantjes J, Dandona R, Macleod-Hall C, McGuinness LA, Schmidt L, Webb RT, Gunnell D (2022) Suicide and self-harm in low- and middle- income countries during the COVID-19 pandemic: a systematic review. PLoS Glob Public Health 2(6):e0000282. https://doi.org/10.1371/journal.pgph.0000282. Accessed 2 Mar 2025

Lewis SP, Collaton J, Pugh RL, Heath NL, Whitley R (2025) The lived experience of self-injury stigma and its psychosocial impact: a thematic analysis. BMC Psychol 13(1):563. https://doi.org/10.1186/s40359-025-02664-6. Accessed 2 Mar 2025

Lloyd B, Blazely A, Phillips L (2018) Stigma towards individuals who self harm: impact of gender and disclosure. J Public Ment Health 17(4):184–194. https://doi.org/10.1108/jpmh-02-2018-0016. Accessed 2 Mar 2025

McManus S, Gunnell D, Cooper C, Bebbington PE, Howard LM, Brugha T, Jenkins R, Hassiotis A, Weich S, Appleby L (2019) Prevalence of non-suicidal self-harm and service contact in England, 2000–14: repeated cross-sectional surveys of the general population. Lancet Psychiatry 6(7):573–581. https://doi.org/10.1016/s2215-0366(19)30188-9. Accessed 2 Mar 2025

Mental Capacity Act 2005, c. 9. Available at: https://www.legislation.gov.uk/ukpga/2005/9

Mental Health Act 1983, c. 1 (1983) London: HMSO

Mental Health Act 2007, c. 12 (2007) London: TSO

Mishara BL, Weisstub DN (2016) The legal status of suicide: a global review. Int J Law Psychiatry 44:54–74. https://doi.org/10.1016/j.ijlp.2015.08.032. Accessed 2 Mar 2025

Moone C, Trenoweth S (2024) Chapter 26: Mental health assessment. In: Wright KM, McKeown M (eds) Essentials of mental health nursing, 2nd edn. SAGE Publications, London

Morris S, Hill S, Brugha T, McManus S (eds.) (2025) Adult Psychiatric Morbidity Survey: Survey of Mental Health and Wellbeing, England, 2023/24. Leeds: NHS England. Available at: https://digital.nhs.uk/data-and-information/publications/statistical/adult-psychiatric-morbidity-survey. Accessed 10 Mar 2026

Mughal F, Burton F, Fletcher H, Lascelles K, O'Connor R, Rae S, Thomson A, Kapur N (2023) New guidance for self-harm: an opportunity not to be missed. Br J Psychiatry 223:501–503. https://doi.org/10.1192/bjp.2023.113. Accessed 2 Mar 2025

National Institute for Health and Care Excellence (2022) Self-harm: assessment, management and preventing recurrence NICE guideline. Available at: https://www.nice.org.uk/guidance/ng225/resources/selfharm-assessment-management-and-preventing-recurrence-pdf-66143837346757. Accessed 2 Mar 2025

NHS Best for You (2026) Self-help and crisis resources. [Online] Cnwl.nhs.uk. Available at: https://www.cnwl.nhs.uk/application/files/6016/4440/0108/Best_Four_You_Poster.png. Accessed 30 Mar 2026

NHS England (2026) Barriers to implementing the Mental Capacity Act in acute settings. Available from: https://www.england.nhs.uk/long-read/guidance-to-support-implementation-of-the-mental-capacity-act-in-acute-trusts-for-adults-with-a-learning-disability/. Accessed 2 Mar 2025

NICE (2025) Self-harm: assessment, management and preventing recurrence (NG225). NICE

Nursing and Midwifery Council (2018) Future nurse: Standards of proficiency for registered nurses. Available at: https://www.nmc.org.uk/standards/standards-for-nurses/standards-of-proficiency-for-registered-nurses/. Accessed 21 July 2026

O'Keeffe S, Suzuki M, Ryan M, Hunter J, McCabe R (2021) Experiences of care for self-harm in the emergency department: comparison of the perspectives of patients, carers and practitioners. BJPsych Open 7(5):e175. https://doi.org/10.1192/bjo.2021.1006. Accessed 2 Mar 2025

POhWER (2022) Independent Mental Health Advocacy (IMHA). Available at: https://www.pohwer.net/independent-mental-health-advocacy-imha. Accessed 21 July 2026

RCPLegal (2023) Case summary: Manchester University Hospitals NHS Foundation Trust v JS. Available at: https://www.rcplegal.co.uk/. Accessed 7 May 2026

Royal College of Psychiatrists (2019) Self-harm and suicide prevention guidance. Available from: https://www.rcpsych.ac.uk/improving-care/nccmh/quality-improvement-programmes/national-suicide-prevention-programme/suicide-prevention-for-those-who-have-self-harmed. Accessed 7 May 2026

Saunders KEA, Hawton K, Fortune S, Farrell S (2012) Attitudes and knowledge of clinical staff regarding people who self-harm: a systematic review. J Affect Disord 139(3):205–216. https://doi.org/10.1016/j.jad.2011.08.024. Accessed 7 May 2026

Stanley B, Brown GK (2012) Safety planning intervention: a brief intervention to mitigate suicide risk. Cogn Behav Pract 19(2):256–264. https://doi.org/10.1016/j.cbpra.2011.01.001. Accessed 7 May 2026

Stanley B, Brown,GK, Karlin B, Kemp JE, VonBergen HA (2008). Safety plan treatment manual to reduce suicide risk: Veteran version. Washington, DC: United States Department of Veterans Affairs, 12

SCIE (2022) Mental Capacity Act: a guide to assessing capacity. Social Care Institute for Excellence, London. Available at: https://www.scie.org.uk/mca/assessment/. Accessed 7 May 2026

SCIE (2026) Overview of the Mental Capacity Act. Social Care Institute for Excellence, London. Available at: https://www.scie.org.uk/mca/introduction/overview/. Accessed 7 May 2026

Scottish Government (2025) Barriers and facilitators to accessing support and services for people who self-harm: a rapid evidence review and survey of practitioner perspectives. Available at: https://www.gov.scot/binaries/content/documents/govscot/publications/research-and-analysis/2025/10/barriers-facilitators-accessing-support-services-people-self-harm-rapid-evidence-review-survey-practitioner-perspectives/documents/barriers-facilitators-accessing-support-services-people-self-harm-rapid-evidence-review-survey-practitioner-perspectives/barriers-facilitators-accessing-support-services-people-self-harm-rapid-evidence-review-survey-practitioner-perspectives/govscot%3Adocument/barriers-facilitators-accessing-support-services-people-self-harm-rapid-evidence-review-survey-practitioner-perspectives.pdf. Accessed 1 Feb 2026

Series L (2025) Written evidence submitted by Dr Lucy series (MHB0022). Available at: https://committees.parliament.uk/writtenevidence/137088/pdf/. Accessed 7 May 2026

The National Confidential Inquiry into Suicide and Safety in Mental Health. Annual Report: UK patient and general population data, 2013–2023. 2026. University of Manchester. Accessed 21 July 2026

The Point of Care Foundation (2026) Schwartz Rounds information. Available from: https://www.pointofcarefoundation.org.uk/our-programmes/schwartz-rounds/. Accessed 7 May 2026

Warrender D (2024) The memoir of a ghost: the invisible plight of mental health nurse education in the United Kingdom following the Nursing and Midwifery Council's move towards genericism. Int J Ment Health Nurs 33:2386–2393. https://doi.org/10.1111/inm.13405. Accessed 7 May 2026

Williams A, Nielson E, Coulson N (2018) 'They aren't all like that': perceptions of clinical services, as told by self-harm online communities. J Health Psychol 25(13–14):2164–2177. Available from: https://pmc.ncbi.nlm.nih.gov/articles/PMC7583449/. Accessed 7 May 2026Wheeler R (2018) Mental Capacity Act and Mental Health Act interactions – legal commentary. Available at: https://www.mentalcapacitylawandpolicy.org.uk/. Accessed 7 May 2026

World Health Organization (2021) Suicide. World Health Organization, Geneva. Available at: https://www.who.int/news-room/fact-sheets/detail/suicide. Accessed 7 May 2026

World Health Organization (2025) Global suicide data. World Health Organization, Geneva. Available at: https://www.who.int/publications/i/item/9789240110069. Accessed 7 May 2026

Challenging Behaviours

Defining: 'Challenging'

Reflective Questions

What behaviour have you seen in your practice which you would classify as challenging behaviour?

What concerns you about working with challenging behaviour?

Emerson (1995) defined challenging behaviours as:

> Culturally abnormal behaviour(s) of such intensity, frequency or duration that the physical safety of the person or others is likely to be placed in serious jeopardy, or behaviour which is likely to seriously limit use of, or result in the person being denied access to, ordinary community services.

More contemptuous definitions may come from The Challenging Behaviour Foundation (2025) which highlights that challenging behaviours are a range of behaviours that some people with learning disabilities may display. This includes hurting others, self-injury, destructive behaviours, eating inedible objects and other behaviours such as spitting or running off. The NHS also agrees that challenging behaviour may include aggression, self-harm, destructiveness and disruptiveness (NHS 2024).

Challenging behaviours are not a diagnosable disorder (Wolkorte et al. 2019). Challenging behaviour as a term has been debated over time, but has replaced many similar terms including abnormal, aberrant, disturbed, dysfunctional and maladaptive (Wolkorte et al. 2019). However, you may also see other terms used in contemporary practice, such as 'behaviour that could be described as challenging', 'behaviours that challenge' and 'behaviours of concern' (McGill 2021).

Whilst we historically view challenging behaviours as related only to learning disabilities, it can indeed occur across the intellectual spectrum. Indeed, challenging

R. Bage, *Mental Health Skills for Adult Nurses & Non-Specialist Healthcare Workers*, https://doi.org/10.1007/978-3-032-32835-9_7

behaviours can be particularly prevalent in those with a psychiatric disorder (Xeniditis et al. 2001).

Case Study

Miss Doyle is a young woman who has a moderate learning disability and sensory processing difficulties. You are working as a practice nurse, and she attends the GP surgery with her support worker for a routine assessment of her asthma.

The waiting area is busy and noisier than normal, with a few poorly toddlers crying. After a short delay, Miss Doyle is coming increasingly distressed. She is rocking in her chair and covering her ears and repeatedly asking when it will be her turn. Her support worker asks the receptionist whether she is going in next, and she is told that unfortunately they have had an emergency and he is now running 30 minutes behind.

Miss Doyle becomes increasing agitated with this and shouts loudly 'I'm not important'. She leaves her seat and pushes past some other service users in the surgery waiting room. Her carer tries to catch her, but she pushes her strongly away and shouts 'I'm going'.

What factors related to miss Doyle's learning disability and sensory processing difficulties may have contributed to her escalating distress?
How could you make this scenario safer in the future?
What adjustments could you have made for Miss Doyle to support her in attending the appointment?

Drivers and Formulation

There are five main reasons why challenging behaviours may be happening which are included in Fig. 1 (Hardy and Joyce 2011).

Attention

When somebody is seeking attention, you may hear staff saying that someone is 'attention seeing' and you may hear this term used in a derogatory or negative way. However, at times of distress, we will all seek the attention of our own loved ones,

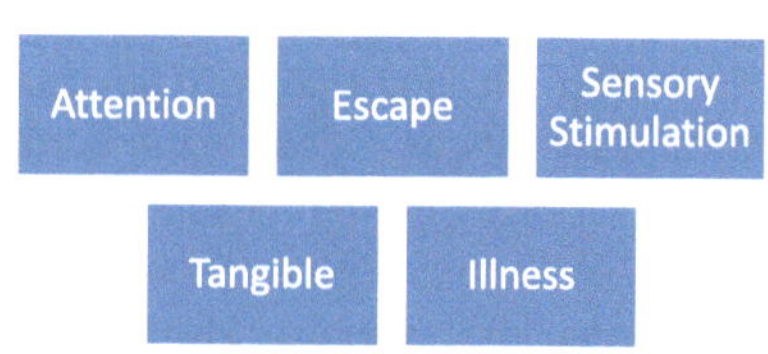

Fig. 1 Challenging behaviours

friends, or strangers. This is a need for social attention from others (Hardy and Joyce 2011).

In mental health, you may see this as when somebody causes deliberate self-injury or in learning disabilities when somebody takes their clothes off. They have learnt that when they demonstrate this behaviour, somebody will come over and give the craved attention.

Case Study

Luca is a resident in a supported living flat. He has a mild learning disability and a history of childhood neglect. He has lived in his current placement for 6 months and is doing well. He presents as generally friendly, but displays occasional challenging behaviour driven by an intense need for reassurance and attention. He often follows staff around, asking if they can talk to him or like him even if staff are occupied or dealing with other situations. When told to wait, Luca can slam doors, throw furniture and shout that no one cares. Luca stops this behaviour quickly once he gains attention.

How can you support Luca to feel valued even when you are busy or unable to give immediate attention?
What strategies might help you stay calm and predictable during repeated or escalating incidents?
How important is consistency between staff responses, and how could you encourage a team to achieve this?

Escape

This is looking at the need to get away from somebody or something. The reasons why might be due to not understanding what is happening and a need to run off because of this. You may see somebody being asked to come to the dinner room for lunch and then running off soon after. They may find that the dinner room is loud, busy, chaotic and overstimulating.

Sensory Stimulation

This is the attempt when we try to stimulate ourselves and to provide our senses with something to formulate. This might be somebody who cuts through deliberate self-injury, or it might be somebody who pulls their hair. This might also be people with a learning disability who hum or sing constantly or prod their eyes to see what happens. Sensory stimulation may be seen most commonly when people do not have the stimulation required (Hardy and Joyce 2011).

Table 1 Challenging behaviour cycle (Challenging Behaviour Foundation 2025)

Stage	Signals
Proactive	Happy, calm, contented
Active	Anxious, aroused, agitated, distressed Fight or flight
Reactive	This is where the incident occurs
Post reactive stage	Calming down, but still opportunity to become reactive again

Tangible

This is where a person gains something due to the behaviours they are exhibiting. This might be something like food or drink, or something such as a toy or book. This happens when you might hear somebody escalating and so to de-escalate the situation you bring the service user a drink (as this has worked previously). The service user had now learnt that if they shout or swear, they might then get something that they want (a drink) (Hardy and Joyce 2011).

Illness

The final reason might be due to illness. For example, somebody may slap their face if they have a headache or toothache. You may see service users pulling or poking at ears if they have an ear infection (Hardy and Joyce 2011).

The Challenging Behaviour Foundation (2025) has offered a useful chart, Table 1, which demonstrates the stages and signals of someone who may be escalating into challenging behaviour.

ABC

You may also find an ABC chart helpful. This is when A = antecedent, B = behaviour and C = consequences (Hardy and Joyce 2011). The purpose of an ABC chart is to identify the link between behaviour and the antecedent and consequences. The aim of this is to understand the function of the behaviours that are being demonstrated (Challenging Behaviours Foundation 2025).

Case Study—Miss Doyle

In Miss Doyle's case, there were some clear triggers within the GP surgery. As with any GP surgery waiting room, they can often be very overstimulating environments. There are often people coming and going, harsh lighting and names being called either by person or electronic system. There is also a level of unpredictability about it—you are not sure if they are running on time, you are not sure who is next, etc.

Equally, she was not aware that an emergency had been brought in and she had been pushed back, with a difficult situation for anyone to manage.

In the future, you would want to consider what would be a better scenario for Miss Doyle. If waiting in such an environment is a known trigger, you might be able to arrange for her to wait in an unoccupied room with her carer. Equally, it might be more appropriate for Miss Doyle to be seen at home if possible.

You would be advised to work proactively with Miss Doyle and her care team to support her to access her health appointments. It is also of great importance that she is not put off from attending health appointments by this experience.

Assessment and Management

Hassiotis and Rudra (2022) proposed a stepped care model for the assessment and management of challenging behaviour. See Fig. 2 which provides a useful visual illustration of the stepped care approach (Hassiotis and Rudra 2022).

This model is a model that does not necessarily function in a linear way and those with challenging behaviours may go up and down steps or skip steps. If there is limited or no response at the lower stage, it is important to act by moving up a step (Hassiotis and Rudra 2022).

Step 1

Behaviours which are low risk of harm to self or others may require limited or no action from carers or family. However, the reasons that may precipitate these behaviours should still be explored. This could involve pain, illness, side-effects of medication, mental illness, constipation or a fluctuating condition such as delirium. It

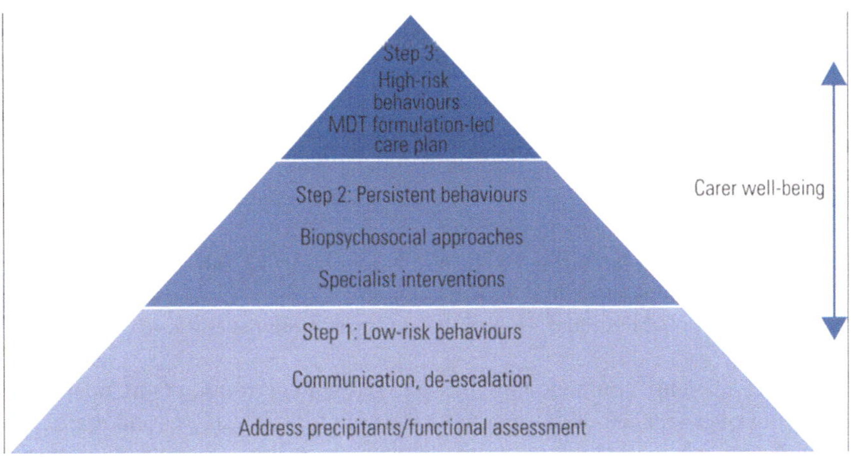

Fig. 2 Stepped care approach for managing behaviours that challenge

may also be appropriate to liaise with GP or primary care for more support (Hassiotis and Rudra 2022).

Low-intensity interventions such as functional assessment may help to understand the reasons for the behaviour. In functional assessment, data is collected from direct observations by carers and then followed by functional assessment. Non-specialised health professionals can be trained to carry out these assessments and to support in the development of a positive behavioural support (PBS) plan (Hassiotis and Rudra 2022).

What Is a PBS Plan?

Gore et al. (2013) write that PBS is a multicomponent framework that is there for developing an understanding of behaviour that challenges. It should be based on a broad assessment of social and physical contexts in which behaviour occurs and used to construct a valid intervention that enhances quality of life.

The key principles of PBS are as follows:

- A PBS plan should consider the person and their life circumstances including physical health and emotional needs. Practitioners should also consider the impact of previous trauma and adverse life events.
- Reduces the likelihood of behaviours that challenge by developing and supporting environments that are supportive and capable of meeting people's needs.
- Is proactive and preventative.
- Aims to teach people new skills to replace behaviours that challenge—these should enhance opportunities for independent, interesting and meaningful lives.
- Input from a range of professionals and multiple evidence-based approaches (Health Education England 2021).

Gore argues that PBS should involve key components—values, theory and evidence base and processes (Gore et al. 2013).

In completing a PBS plan you should:

Provide a clear description of behaviours of concern (including if these behaviours are sequenced or clustered together)
The identification of events, times and situations that predict when behaviour may or may not occur and how these match with a person's daily routines
Identification of the consequences that maintain the behaviours (purposes or functions that the behaviours may serve)
Summary statements that describe specific behaviours, the situations in which they occur and consequences that may maintain it
Direct observational data that support the summary statements (Gore et al. 2013)

A research study completed in 2021 worked with children, young people and parents to co-design a toolkit to promote the use of PBS strategies and reasonable adjustments when a child with intellectual disabilities or autistic spectrum attends a general hospital for a clinical procedure. Following this work, they were able to develop 'My Hospital Guide' for use by others (Health Research Authority 2020).

Step 2

If step one is not successful, manualised interventions can be completed by trained professionals. This could involve therapies such as CBT or mindfulness, or more advanced therapies include eye-movement desensitisation and reprocessing (EMDR). These are normally delivered by people working within learning disability services or services within NHS talking therapies (Hassiotis and Rudra 2022).

Step 3

The final step is for the most high-risk situations who are not responding to step 1 or 2. These cases require an in-depth multidisciplinary team formulation for a more detailed understanding of problems and interventions. At this point, inpatient admission or respite care may be considered (Hassiotis and Rudra 2022).

Prevention: Environment & Communication

Environmental factors can refer to physical factors and additional physical factors and a quality of life (Hardy and Joyce 2011). It may help us to think about the environment in three categories—physical, interpersonal and programmatic.

Physical
Foundations of de-escalation
Crisis response
Staff wellbeing and emotional resilience
LD/Autism Considerations

Reflective Questions
What is your confidence level in working with service users who have a learning disability or autism diagnosis?

Historically, antipsychotics have been used to 'manage' behaviours that people have found challenging (de Kujiper et al. 2022). Stopping over medication of people with a learning disability and autistic people (STOMP) is a national NHS England work programme to stop the inappropriate use of long-term psychotropic medication. People with a learning disability are 16× more likely, and autistic people 7× more likely to be prescribed an antipsychotic than the general population (NHS England 2025a).

Mencap (2010) produced the 'Getting it Right Charter' which looks at people with a learning disability getting an equal right to healthcare. As part of this charter, nine different pledges can be made:

- Make sure that hospital passports are available and used within your environment.
- Make sure that all our staff understand and apply the principles of mental capacity laws.
- Appoint a learning disability liaison nurse within our hospitals.
- Make sure every eligible person with a learning disability can have an annual health check.
- Provide ongoing learning disability awareness training for all staff.
- Listen to, respect and involve families and carers.
- Provide practical support and information to families and carers.
- Provide information that is accessible for people with a learning disability.
- Display the Getting it right principles for everyone to see.

In the latest report, republished in 2026, adults with a learning disability die on average 19.5 years younger than the general population. This means that the median age of adults with a learning disability to die is just 62.5 years old. Avoidable deaths have, thankfully, declined since 2021, but the rate of avoidable death for adults with a learning disability is nearly double the rate compared to the general population. The most common avoidable deaths in this group are influenza, pneumonia, heart diseases and cerebrovascular diseases (Strydom et al. 2026).

A proportion of people with a learning disability will present with behaviour that could be classified as challenging. In adults, that figure is about 10–15%, and most common in males, people with autism and those with a more severe disability (National Centre for Mental Health 2026). These behaviours may include aggression, self-injury, property destruction or outbursts (Lim 2024).

Health and Care Passport

The health and care passport is designed to be a simple way to give health and social care professional's information about a person with a learning disability or autism to ensure they get the right care and treatment. It should make it clear whether reasonable adjustments are required, and what these need to be. People with a learning disability can either complete these independently or with support from family or carers (NHS England 2024a). Some people may have a copy saved online or they may have a printed copy (NHS England 2024a).

If you are working with a person with a learning disability, it is important to make sure they are kept up to date and reviewed regularly.

Reasonable Adjustments

The Equality Act (2010) states all organisations, including those in health and social care, must take steps to remove the barriers individuals face because of disability. You can help to do this by making, often small, changes to the way that you care for people. These changes are called reasonable adjustments (NHS England 2025b). Some reasonable adjustments that you could make to people with a learning disability or autism could be:

- Making sure you provide leaflets and letters in plain English or easy-read letters.
- Having a quiet space for somebody to wait for an appointment.
- Making sure you document whether a person has a health and care passport.
- Ensuring you are using any communication aids which a person might need.
- Sending information ahead of an appointment about what will happen within an appointment.

The QS101 quality standard from NICE (NICE 2019) highlights support and services for children, young people and adults with a learning disability (or a learning disability and autism) and behaviour that challenges. It contains 12 quality statements which need to be met to demonstrate high quality care for this cohort.

Quality Statement 1: Lead Commissioner

This statement looks further at having a lead person to oversee strategic commissioning of services for people with learning disabilities. This aims to bring together commissioning across health, social care and education for children, young people and adults. This aims to both simplify the system and to ensure a positive experience for a person with learning disabilities and their family and carers.

Quality Statement 2: Annual Health Check

This standard looks at the importance of people with a learning disability having an annual health check from their GP. This allows for underlying physical health problems to be identified at an early stage. It argues that unrecognised physical illness may lead to pain or discomfort which then will potentially lead on to behaviour that challenges.

Quality Statement 3: Initial Assessment of Behaviour That Challenges

This looks at an early assessment to identify possible triggers, environmental factors and functions of challenging behaviour. This assessment will help identify and seek action on the factors that may be leading people to behave in a way that challenges.

Quality Statement 4: Named Lead Practitioner

This standard looks at the importance of people who have a learning disability and behaviour that challenges having a named lead practitioner. This aims to co-ordinate support and make sure services are working together.

Quality Statement 5: Involving Families and Carers

This statement looks at the importance of involving people who are key figures in a person's life in developing a person's care and support plan. This should involve guidance on how to prevent or respond to a crisis.

Quality Statement 6: Parent-Training Programmes

This quality statement identified that parents or carers of children aged under 12 years with a learning disability and behaviour that challenges should be offered a parent-training programme.

Quality Statement 7: Personalised Daily Activities

This quality statement identified that people with a learning disability and behaviour that challenges take part in personalised daily activities. High levels of behaviour that challenges have been reported in institutions that offer relatively limited activities. Ensuring that people with a learning disability have a planned daily activity planner will reduce rates of behaviour that challenge.

Quality Statement 8: Services in the Community

People with a learning disability and behaviour that challenges have access to specialist behavioural support in the community. Insufficient community support can impact quality of life for people with a learning disability and behaviour that challenges and can prevent or delay discharge or transition.

Quality Statement 9: Housing

People with a learning disability and behaviour that challenges face barriers to choosing where they live. This statement highlights the importance of people being able to choose where and how they live.

Quality Statement 10: Review of Restrictive Interventions

People with a learning disability and behaviour that challenges should have a documented review every time a restrictive intervention is used. Restrictive interventions should be used as a last resort and based on the principles of using the least restrictive intervention necessary.

Quality Statement 11: Use of Medication

People with a learning disability and behaviour that challenges should only receive antipsychotic medication as part of a treatment that includes psychosocial interventions. Antipsychotic medication is the most frequently used drug for people with a learning disability and behaviour that challenges, often in the absence of a diagnosis of a mental health problem.

Quality Statement 12: Review of Medication
People with a learning disability and behaviour that challenges have a multidisciplinary review of their antipsychotics medication 12 weeks after starting and then at least every 6 months.

The Role of the Learning Disability Liaison Nurse

Reflective Questions
Do you know if you have access to a learning disability liaison nurse?
Do you know their role or remit within your local trust or services?

There have long been concerns about the care of people with a learning disability within acute care settings. The learning disability liaison nurse was a role established to ensure that additional specialist support is available for service users, carers, families and general healthcare practitioners (Brown et al. 2011). The role is a complex role, and varies by location, but some of the most important aspects of a learning disability liaison nurse could be summarised as—clinical service user care, education and practice development, and strategic organisational developments (Brown et al. 2011).

One of the other key roles about learning disability liaison nurses is their ability to support with capacity assessments. A Health Services Safety Investigations Body Report (2023) found that in acute hospital inpatient environments, there was variation in staff understanding and application of the mental capacity act in the care of people with a learning disability.

Personality Disorders

Whilst positive behaviour plans have been implemented successfully in learning disabilities, there have been challenges in doing this for mental health services.

One of the challenges has been around observation. Many of those who present with challenging behaviours in learning disability services live with higher levels of support which has made observations and assessments a very possible option. Many of these observations rely on carers and family to support, and then their involvement is required when implementing the PBS plans. However, in people who have a diagnosis of personality disorder, they are often living independently and often have limited to no support. Indeed, mental health services are often set up to reduce support over time and discharge from active services. This makes direct observations and observations during the implementation stage of a PBS plan much more challenging. This then puts a greater emphasis on reflection in the PBS development and implementation process (Brown et al. 2017).

Brown et al. (2017) developed a strategy to include PBS within their own NHS services using a traffic light system (green: okay, amber: build up, red: incident, blue: cool down). It allowed service users to reflect on their own behaviours both internally and externally.

Learning from Incidents

One of the challenges within learning disability services is the lack of learning disability nurses. Recent analysis from the Royal College of Nursing found there has been a huge collapse in the number of student learning disability nurses. There has been a 36% drop in acceptances to learning disability nursing courses between 2015 and 2023 and only 2% of all nursing course acceptances were for learning disability courses in 2023 (RCN 2024). It is interesting to consider the reasons behind this. Many learning disability services are split between social and healthcare services making jobs less clear for potential candidates. Equally, universities may only offer the course if there is demand from local services, and this simply may not be the case in many of our regions. It certainly should be a great worry that there are simply not the learning disability nurses entering the workforce.

Oliver McGowan

Oliver McGowan was 18 at the time of his death and was an inpatient at North Bristol NHS Trust. He was a young man, who died from a relatively rare condition, known as neuroleptic malignancy syndrome relating to the use of antipsychotics which his parents had not consented to. Oliver had previously had a poor reaction to antipsychotics and his family had made this clear (Oliver McGowan, n.d.)

The Oliver McGowan Mandatory Training on learning disabilities and autism is named after OIiver McGowan. The Health and Care Act 2022 introduced a statutory requirement that CQC registered providers must ensure that their staff receive learning disability and autism training. The Oliver McGowan Mandatory Training has become the standardised training developed to meet this requirement and is the preferred training for most health care providers (Obe 2022; HEE 2022).

Myles Scriven

Myles Scriven was a 31-year-old man who died at Huddersfield Royal Infirmary in April 2023 from a treatable blood clot in his leg. An Inquest into his death found there was multiple missed opportunities to save his life with Calderdale Royal Hospital and GP practice. There were limited reasonable adjustments may despite the fact he had a learning disability and was autistic, and family had flagged that he would require support to make medical decisions. The coroner found that a lack of adjustment for Myle's learning disability and autism and neglect contributed to his death. He commented that clinicians were 'blind' to his needs (Courts and Tribunals Judiciary 2025).

Ethics, Rights and Restrictive Practices

Learning Disabilities

There have been plenty of recent news articles and media coverage of restrictive practices that are continued to be used in the learning difficulties sector. We should all consider the use of long-term inappropriate inpatient beds for people with learning disabilities or autism as a failure in our health and social care. Joint work between Mencap and ITV News found that approximately £534 million is being spent on inpatient beds for just over 2000 people with a learning disability and autistic people in England (Mencap 2024).

The changes in the Mental Health Act (moving from 1983 to 2025) mean that people with a learning disability or autism will no longer be able to be detained under Section 3 of the Act, unless they have a co-occurring mental health disorder (NHS Confederation 2025).

Personality Disorders

Equally, challenges remain in placements for those with personality disorders. As Harding et al. (2020) writes, people with a personality disorder can often be moved to specialist personality disorders, a term where there is no clear safeguard or standards and are essentially locked rehabilitation units, and people are held under the Mental Health Act in very restrictive environments. Harding et al. (2020) discusses these units as a place for outsourcing risk. The cost of these units, which are largely private, are staggeringly high and it could be argued to be a poor option for people with a personality disorder diagnosis.

Key Learning Points

We must change our mindsets to consider challenging behaviour as a method of communication, and not 'bad behaviour'. When presented with challenging behaviour, we must start to think about unmet needs, physical ill health, pain or sensory overwhelm. We must ensure that we are not judging.

We must consider the environment that the service user is in. Environment can often lead to overload, and we should consider how we can change the environment to ensure people are not overloaded.

Medications continue to be overused in services, especially learning disability and autism services. Nurses and other health professionals play a key role in advocating for non-pharmacological services.

Restrictive practices should always be the last resort, and this is supported by national policies and ethics frameworks. By planning in advance, and by providing holistic person-centred care, we can significantly reduce restrictive practices used across health services.

Every clinician should have knowledge of some of the high-profile cases involving learning disability, mental health and autism cases. We should learn from previous experiences and reflect to ensure systems are better in the future.

Conclusion

Challenging behaviours must be understood not as problems with an individual, but as an expression of unmet need. This might range from physical pain or sensory overload to trauma, fear, frustration, or environmental mismatch. Throughout this chapter, we have explored how behaviours arise within a complex interaction of biological, psychological, social and environmental factors, and how a holistic, person-centred formulation enables practitioners to respond with compassion rather than judgement. Discussion of models and frameworks such as the ABC model, stress-vulnerability approach and Positive Behaviour Support (PBS), has helped develop knowledge and hopefully confidence in your own skill set and ability. These approaches encourage us to move beyond simply reacting to behaviours and instead seek to understand the meaning and purpose behind them.

This chapter has highlighted that prevention is key. Understanding environments, communication styles, routines and triggers can help us identify ways to reduce distress before situations escalate. Equally, we understand the importance of involving family members and carers who are often highly knowledgeable about the individuals they support and can provide valuable insight into needs, preferences, and behavioural patterns. We have also been able to see where systems and practice have failed—such as the cases of Oliver McGowan and Myles Scriven—and I hope we can all recognise why healthcare and social care services must continue striving to do better. These cases remind us of the devastating consequences that can occur when communication, listening and person-centred care are absent.

As clinicians, we always need to stay curious. We need to ask questions to make sure we fully understand the experiences and needs of those we support. We need to remain reflective in our practice and willing to challenge our own assumptions, attitudes and responses. We need the drive to understand what is behind the behaviours that we are seeing, rather than focussing solely on the behaviour itself. The skills and principles outlined throughout this chapter are central not only to good practice in managing challenging behaviours, but also to ensuring that we remain compassionate, therapeutic and person-centred practitioners who promote dignity, safety and inclusion in all aspects of care.

References

Brown JF, Brown MZ and Dibiasio P (2017) Treating individuals with personality disorder using positive behaviour support: clinical applications in community mental health services. IJPBS 7(2):24–35

Brown M, MacArthur J, McKechanie A, Mack S, Hayes M, Fletcher J (2011) Learning Disability Liaison Nursing Services in south-east Scotland: a mixed-methods impact and outcome study. J Intellect Disabil Res 56(12):1161–1174. https://doi.org/10.1111/j.1365-2788.2011.01511.x. Accessed 7 May 2026

Courts and Tribunals Judiciary (2025) Myles Scriven (1): Prevention of Future Deaths Report. Available at: https://www.judiciary.uk/prevention-of-future-death-reports/myles-scriven-prevention-of-future-deaths-report/. Accessed 22 July 2026

de Kuijper G, de Haan J, Deb S Shankar R (2022) Withdrawing antipsychotics for challenging behaviours in adults with intellectual disabilities: experiences and views of experts by experience. Int J Environ Res Public Health 19(23):15637. https://doi.org/10.3390/ijerph192315637

Emerson E (1995) cited in Emerson, E (2001, 2nd edition): Challenging Behaviour: Analysis and intervention in people with learning disabilities. Cambridge University Press

Gore NJ, McGill P, Toogood S, Allen D, Hughes JC, Baker P, Hastings RP, Noone SJ, Denne LD (2013) Definition and scope for positive behavioural support. Int J Posit Behav Support 3(2):14–23

Hardy S, Joyce T (eds.) (2011) Challenging Behaviour and People with Learning Disabilities: A Handbook. Brighton: Pavilion Publishing

Harding K, Poole R, Robinson C (2020) The outsourcing of risk: out-of-area placements for individuals diagnosed with personality disorder in the UK. Lancet Psychiatry 7(9):730–731. https://doi.org/10.1016/S2215-0366(20)30148-6. Accessed 7 May 2026

Hassiotis A. Rudra S (2022) Behaviours that challenge in adults with intellectual disability: overview of assessment and management. BJPsych Adv 28(6):393–400. https://doi.org/10.1192/bja.2022.28. Accessed 21 July 2026

Health Education England (2021) The key messages about Positive Behaviour Support. Available at: https://www.hee.nhs.uk/sites/default/files/documents/The%20key%20messages%20about%20Positive%20Behaviour%20Support_0.pdf. Accessed 21 July 2026

Health Education England (2022) The Oliver McGowan Mandatory Training on Learning Disability and Autism. Available at: https://www.hee.nhs.uk/our-work/learning-disability/current-projects/oliver-mcgowan-mandatory-training-learning-disability-autism. Accessed 21 July 2026

Health Research Authority (2020) Positive Behaviour Support Toolkit for C/YP attending hospital v1. [Online] Health Research Authority. Available at: https://www.hra.nhs.uk/planning-and-improving-research/application-summaries/research-summaries/positive-behaviour-support-toolkit-for-cyp-attending-hospital-v1/. Accessed 30 Mar 2026

Lim M-A (2024) Managing behaviours of concern in adults with learning disabilities. The Estia Centre Blog, South London and Maudsley NHS Foundation Trust, 24 January. Available at: https://slam.nhs.uk/estiacentre-blog/managing-behaviours-of-concern-in-adults-with-learning-disabilities-4326. Accessed 7 May 2026

McGill P (2021) Understanding challenging behaviour: part 1. [Online] Information Sheet. Available at: https://www.challengingbehaviour.org.uk/wp-content/uploads/2021/02/001-Understanding-Challenging-Behaviour-Part-1.pdf. Accessed 7 May 2026

Mencap (2010) Getting it right charter: See the person, not the disability. Available at: https://www.mencap.org.uk. Accessed 21 July 2026.

Mencap (2024) Over half a billion pounds a year is spent locking up people with a learning disability and / or autistic people in mental health hospitals in England. Available at: https://www.mencap.org.uk/press-release/over-half-billion-pounds-year-spent-locking-people-learning-disability-and-or. Accessed 21 July 2026

National Centre for Mental Health (2026) Learning disability, mental health and challenging behaviour [online]. Cardiff: NCMH. Available from: https://www.ncmh.info/wp-content/uploads/2016/04/Web-2026-NCMH-Learning-disability-mental-health-and-challenging-behaviour-A5-leaflet.pdf. Accessed 21 July 2026

NHS (2024) How to deal with challenging behaviour in adults. Available at: https://www.nhs.uk/social-care-and-support/practical-tips-if-you-care-for-someone/how-to-deal-with-challenging-behaviour-in-adults/. Accessed 21 July 2026

NHS Confederation (2025) The Mental Health Act 2025: what you need to know. [Online] NHS Confederation. Available at: https://www.nhsconfed.org/publications/mental-health-act-2025-what-you-need-know. Accessed 7 May 2026

NHS England (2024a) Health and care passport—plain English. [Online] England.nhs.uk. Available at: https://www.england.nhs.uk/long-read/health-and-care-passport-plain-english/#what-is-a-health-and-care-passport. Accessed 7 May 2026

NHS England (2024b) The Oliver McGowan Mandatory training in learning disability and autism. [Online] Health Education England. Available at: https://www.hee.nhs.uk/our-work/learning-disability/current-projects/oliver-mcgowan-mandatory-training-learning-disability-autism. Accessed 7 May 2026

NHS England (2025a) Stopping over medication of people with a learning disability and autistic people (STOMP) and supporting treatment and appropriate medication in paediatrics (STAMP). Available at: https://www.england.nhs.uk/learning-disabilities/improving-health/stomp-stamp/. Accessed 21 July 2026

NHS England (2025b) Reasonable adjustments. Available at: https://www.england.nhs.uk/learning-disabilities/improving-health/reasonable-adjustments/ Accessed 21 July 2026

NICE (2019) Overview | Learning disability: behaviour that challenges | Quality standards | NICE. [Online] www.nice.org.uk. Available at: https://www.nice.org.uk/guidance/qs101. Accessed 7 May 2026

Obe F (2022) Independent review into Thomas Oliver McGowan's LeDeR process. Phase two. Chair on behalf of Oliver's Independent Panel for NHS England and NHS Improvement. [Online]. Available at: https://www.england.nhs.uk/wp-content/uploads/2020/10/Independent-Review-into-Thomas-Oliver-McGowans-LeDeR-Process-phase-two-_20-October-2020.pdf. Accessed 7 May 2026

Oliver McGowan (n.d.) Oliver McGowan. Available at: https://www.olivermcgowan.org/. Accessed 21 July 2026

Royal College of Nursing (2024) New RCN analysis reveals devastating collapse in learning disability nursing workforce. [Online] The Royal College of Nursing. Available at: https://www.rcn.org.uk/news-and-events/Press-Releases/new-rcn-analysis-reveals-devastating-collapse-in-learning-disability-nursing-workforce. Accessed 7 May 2026

Strydom A, White P, Heslop P, Blair P, Chinn D, Glover G, Gray R, Scior K, colleagues (2026) Learning from lives and deaths – people with a learning disability and autistic people (LeDeR): Annual report 2023 (revised January 2026). London: NHS England. Available at: https://data.parliament.uk/DepositedPapers/Files/DEP2025-0630/LeDeR_2023_Report_28012026_REVISED_VERSION.pdf. Accessed 21 July 2026

The Challenging Behaviour Foundation (2025) Formal definitions of challenging behaviour. Available at: https://www.challengingbehaviour.org.uk/learning-disability-files/Formal-Definitions-of-Challenging-Behaviour-.pdf. Accessed 21 July 2026

Xeniditis K, Russell A Murphy D. (2001) Management of people with challenging behaviour. Adv Psychiatr Treat 7(2):109–116. https://doi.org/10.1192/apt.7.2.109. Accessed 21 July 2026.

Wolkorte R, van Houwelingen I, Kroezen M (2019) Challenging behaviours: views and preferences of people with intellectual disabilities. J Appl Res Intellect Disabil 32(6):1421–1427. https://doi.org/10.1111/jar.12631. Accessed 7 May 2026

Healthcare Environments

Why Here? Pathways & Politics

Care pathways first began in the USA during the 1980s within managed care, with the idea coming over to the UK in the early 1990s (Evans-Lacko et al. 2018). Care pathways can be defined as:

> a tool and a concept that embed guidelines, protocols, and locally agreed, evidence-based, patient-centred, best practice, into everyday use for the individual patient. In addition, and uniquely to ICPS (integrated care pathways), they record deviations from planned care in the form of variances. (Whittle 2007)

You may know some pathways within your own service. A popular pathway is the 'Model Acute Pathway: standards for care of acutely unwell service users in their first 72 hours in hospital' (NHS England 2026). Pathways in mental health services are used in the same way. The NHS Long Term Plan set out a plan to create a comprehensive crisis pathway in every area. It worked on developing comprehensive and accessible local crisis care pathways—such as adult crisis and home treatment teams, crisis alternatives and simplifying access to urgent mental health support (NHS England 2019).

A Hertfordshire Project NHS Foundation Trust project focused on delivering safer care pathways in mental health services. It focussed on acute mental health care and dementia care pathways across the Easter region's five mental health trusts. It aimed to improve service user safety by addressing teamwork and communication uses that impact safety and effectiveness of care, and service user experience. The evaluation showed that the intervention was effective in supporting the sites to make positive changes to clinical pathways, although barriers involved included maintaining momentum and CQC inspections (The Health Foundation n.d.).

R. Bage, *Mental Health Skills for Adult Nurses & Non-Specialist Healthcare Workers*, https://doi.org/10.1007/978-3-032-32835-9_8

Unwarranted Variation in Mental Health Care

Health care can vary in different ways due to quality, equity, outcomes and the money spent. Some variation is always to be expected and linked to service user preference or levels of illness. However, some is 'unwarranted' and cannot be explained by the same reasons (Gov.uk 2015).

Lord Carter's report, published in 2018, highlighted unwarranted variation in mental health services. Clinical Commissioning Groups commission some mental health services against detailed and different specifications leading to unwarranted variations. There was also noted to be unwarranted variation within direct care time per clinical day in community services and the number of duration of contacts (NHS England 2019).

A&E

Case Study

Alex is a university graduate, who arrives at A + E accompanied by a friend who is worried about sudden changes in his behaviour. Over the last week, Alex has reported intense anxiety, difficulty sleeping and hopelessness linked to work restricting and work pressure. Earlier that day, Alex disclosed to his friends that he had thoughts of self-harm and not feeling safe in his flat. His friend brought him to A + E due to his concerns.

On arrival, Alex is clearly distressed. He is pacing in the waiting room and highly tearful. Alex's friend says he has been struggling in the bright lights of the waiting room and with the unexpected noises. Alex states he feels 'overwhelmed' and he just wants things to 'shut up'. Triage staff note some suicidal ideation, increasing agitation and no current substance misuse.

What immediate risks would you assess when Alex is in the department?

What observations and physical assessments are essential before the mental health review?

How would you approach Alex to help-de-escalate their visible distress in a noisy, overstimulation environment?

The proportion of people attending A + E for a named mental health disorder is thought to be relatively small (Buchanan 2024). However, in 2023–24 saw more than 80,000 people who presented with mental health crises experience more than a 12-hour wait in emergency departments (Mason et al. 2025). Of all mental health presentations in A + E between April 2024 and March 2025, 50% involved self-injurious behaviours and/or suicidal intent or behaviour and 4% involved complex behaviour and hallucinations (Taylor 2026).

People who attend A + E for mental health complaints are more likely to receive no treatment or written advice compared to those who present with other symptoms.

Approximately 40% of people who attend A + E with mental health presentation had a treatment recorded which included cardiac monitoring, intravenous cannulas or administration of medication (Taylor 2026).

International evidence has suggested that mental health patient's long waits in A + E departments are linked with increased restraint and higher use of sedation (Lee et al. 2023). A further systematic review suggested that long waits in A + E departments lead to an increasing level of agitation and distress (Austin et al. 2024).

If we think about our own experiences attending A + E as a patient, it can often be an overwhelming and unpleasant experience. The overwhelming noise of hospital equipment and chatter. The lights, often industrial and white in style. The unpredictability of waiting times, and lack of clear order, can make many overwhelmed and stressed.

In traditional A + E departments, much of the work navigating physical and mental health is done by liaison psychiatry services. Liaison mental health services are there to assess service users, manage risks, and distinguish the symptoms between physical health and mental health (Taylor 2026). Liaison services work across A + E departments, wards and outpatient clinics. They work as multidisciplinary teams to care for those who acute mental health crisis and to help those with pre-existing mental illness who are physically unwell. They also support those with neuropsychiatric symptoms, alcohol and substance misuse, and medically unexplained symptoms (Sampson et al. 2022).

NHS England signed the Crisis Care Concordant and began a piece of work to ensure 24/7 access to the right services for those with mental health crisis. This included a nearly £250 million investment in urgent and emergency mental health liaison in acute hospitals, and community crisis care (NHS England 2014). The aim is for as many services as possible to achieve 'core 24' status, which means they provide a liaison service that is 24 hours a day, 7 days a week.

The 10-Year Health Plan aimed to increase more specialist mental health crisis centres. In 2025, specialist mental health crisis centres begun to be opened in what will be an NHS trial over a decade. Initial pilot sites were Avon and Wiltshire, Blackpool, Lincolnshire, East London, Leicestershire, and Camden and Islington in North London (BBC 2025). The aim of these environments is to allow service users presenting with mental health crisis to avoid long waits within emergency departments (BBC 2025). However, Dr. Lade Smith of the Royal College of Psychiatrists highlighted their concerns that standalone A + E departments may lead to physical health may be missed or inadequately treated. They highlighted concern regarding communication barriers and delays if service users are presenting with both physical health and mental health problems (RCPsych 2025).

Mental Health A + E and Mental Health Urgent Assessment Centres

People with a mental health problem attend A + E in a period of real crisis, and often at a period of last resort. Mental health attendances at A + E Departments are complex and thought to make up about 3% of people in A + E at any one moment. About 50% involve self-injurious and/or suicidal intent and behaviour, and around 35% involve complex behaviours (Nuffield Trust 2026). People who attend A + E are most likely to receive no treatment in A + E or just receive written advice, compared to those with other complaints (Nuffield Trust 2026).

In 2025, NHS England announced the planned opening of 15 mental health crisis assessment centres to provide care in the right place for service users and avoid them waiting in A + E for significant periods of time. A + E has also been agreed to not be the most appropriate place for people in crisis. The aim of these units was to offer access timely access to specialist support (NHS England 2025).

However, there has been concern about this approach to mental health. Dr. Lade Smith raised concerns that separating care increases the risk that a physical health need may be missed or inadequately treated. However, Dr. Smith discusses that these units can be useful when they are colocated with A + E Departments, such as the case of Hull University Hospital (RCPsych 2025). She also raises that this strategy of mental healthcare risks increasing the stigma and divide between mental and physical health services (RCPsych 2025).

Task

1. Where is your nearest MUHAC or Mental Health A + E Department?
2. If you had a service user in crisis, does your local services have an alternative to A + E?

The Mental Health Urgent Assessment Centre (MUHAC) Trial in Lincolnshire

The MUHAC within Lincolnshire Partnership Foundation Trust was a trial of a new service delivery model which aimed to support people in mental health crisis. The aim of the trial was to reduce system pressures across the whole of Lincolnshire health service, by directing people away from emergency departments and into other colocated Mental Health services.

The MUHAC addition involved an evaluation using qualitative and quantitative analysis of data and analysis of service user and staff surveys and interviews. The analysis of this showed this development had been well-received by service users and staff with approximately 85% that it was a better alternative for service users in crisis. There was also evidence to suggest that this had been a cost-effective approach with a reduction in inpatient attendances and relapses. When these cost savings are scaled to the Midlands region, these benefits could reach over £14.4 million annually (Edge Health 2025).

Acute Services

In 2024, there were 17,836 mental health beds within the UK, which is the lowest level since 2010. Bed occupancy remains consistently over the recommended 85%, which can lead to longer waits for beds (Gilburt and Mallorie 2024). The average length of stay in an acute mental health bed has increased in recent years, with the latest data giving an average length of stay of 39 days.

There has been a longstanding relationship between NHS mental health services and the independent sector, far more than seen in general services (Gilburt 2025). Providing NHS-funded care is by far the biggest segment of the independent market value—approximately 92% of their market value is generated from either NHS or local authority funding streams (LaingBuisson 2024).

Mental health service users continue to experience frequent out-of-area placements, the number of which have not declined since 2018 (Gilburt and Mallorie 2024). In October 2023, 59% of those in out-of-area placements had to travel more than 100 km from their home (Gilburt and Mallorie 2024).

Types of Beds

In Table 1, the beds available in mental health services can be seen (NHS England Digital, n.d).

Table 1 Mental health beds

National code	Bed type category	National code definition
200	Acute adult mental health care	These are adult acute beds for working age (18–65) adults. Service users may be admitted to acute mental health wards informally or under the Mental Health Act. The expectation is that these beds are now meeting the single sex accommodation standards.
201	Acute older adult mental health care (organic and functional)	Older adult beds are provided for over 65s. These are typically, although not always, split into two different types of care: Organic mental illness Functional mental illness
202	Adult psychiatric intensive care units (PICU)	A PICU is a psychiatric inpatient unit which are secure—this means they are locked. Staffing levels are normally higher than on acute wards, and this patient group cannot usually be managed safely on acute inpatient wards. Service users in PICU's are normally detained under the Mental Health Act. PICU's are normally for working age adults.

(continued)

Table 1 (continued)

National code	Bed type category	National code definition
203	Adult eating disorders	A bed designed for the treatment of psychiatric illness associated with eating disorders. This will normally have a multidisciplinary team who are specially trained to manage the acute period of an eating disorder.
204	Mother and baby units	These are specialist beds which focus on the care of mothers and their babies. Perinatal units are for both mother and baby and avoid the need to split mum and baby in the important postnatal period.
205	Acute mental health units for adults with a learning disability and/or autism	Adult acute mental health inpatient services are specifically for people who have a learning disability and for autistic people. This is a specialist mental health service. An admission to this unit will only take place when: The person has a learning disability or is autistic They meet the criteria for admission to an acute mental health hospital Sufficient reasonable adjustments cannot practicably be made to the physical environment or staffing of a mental health inpatient service.
206	Adult low secure	Low secure units deliver intensive support who have challenging behaviour in the context of a serious mental illness and who required added layer of security. Service users will normally be detained under the Mental Health Act and may be restricted on legal grounds.
207	Adult medium secure	Medium secure units are normally entered by court, although some come from general mental health services. All are detained under the Mental Health Act. They may also move to medium secure service by transfer from either low or high secure services due to changing needs.
208	Adult high secure	Service users enter high secure care from court, and all will be detained under the Mental Health Act. For example, Rampton Hospital, Nottinghamshire.
209	Adult neuropsychiatry/ acquired brain injury	Neuropsychiatry and acquired brain injury beds are complex inpatient beds for people who have experienced brain injury.
210	Adult personality disorder	Personality disorder inpatient beds offer a very structured environment designed to promote recovery. Services offer a range of therapies alongside additional interventions. A prior diagnosis of personality disorder and associated mental health needs is needed before admission.
211	Adult mental health services for the deaf	These beds offer assessment, treatment and interventions for those who behavioural, mental illness and psychological problems in adults with severe and profound hearing loss. Care is provided by a mixture of deaf and hearing professionals supported by BSL interpreters.

(continued)

Table 1 (continued)

National code	Bed type category	National code definition
212	Adult mental health rehabilitation	Low secure rehabilitation services are hospital based and provide care for service users who have been involved in offending or challenging behaviours. All service users are detained under the Mental Health Act. The usual aim of the treatment is to move on to a high dependency or community rehabilitation unit.
213	Adult Mental Health Rehabilitation for adults with a learning disability and/or autism	Service users who need this kind of facility will be highly symptomatic, with multiple or severe co-morbid conditions, significant risk histories and challenging behaviours. Most will be detained under the MHA. Around 20% will have had forensic admissions. The focus is on thorough ongoing assessment, maximising benefits from medication, engagement, reducing challenging behaviours and reengaging with families and communities. These units have a major role in repatriating patients from secure services and out-of-area placements to local services and, ultimately, to local community living.

What Are Acute Inpatient Units Like?

Reflective Questions

Would it worry you working on a mental health ward?

What things might you be apprehensive about when working on a mental health ward?

Many people have questions about what acute inpatient units are like. A recent conversation with a student adult nurse brought this into my attention, when they asked, 'are mental health wards scary?'.

The truth is that mental health wards are much like any other wards. It often depends on the mix of service users on the ward at the time. Some are mixed sex, although thankfully we are moving towards having single sex wards wherever possible. They often contain a significant amount of laughter, fun and jokes. I fondly remember the time service users on the ward I was working on having time to go to the beach, the castle and strawberry picking on long weekends when ward rounds were not on. However, at times, wards can be very traumatising places for our service users. As discussed earlier in this book, wards can often retraumatise our service users. They can be loud, unpredictable and will contain very unwell service users. At times, this does require people to be restrained physically or secluded.

There has been significant work happened recently to improve the quality of mental health wards. Since 2000, all new-build acute mental health units have been required to have single bedrooms, ideally with ensuites. The Care Quality

Commission (CQC) has identified that service users and carers have negative opinions of shared sleeping arrangements, due to concerns around disturbed sleep, lack of privacy and risk to personal safety (CQC 2019).

Crisis and Home Treatment Teams

Crisis and Home Treatment Teams (CRHT) in mental health services manage service users with risk to self and risk to others in the community (Raja et al. 2024). They also provide rapid assessments for individuals experiencing mental health crisis and offers an alternative to in-patient mental health services (Lloyd-Evans and Johnson 2019). All areas should now be providing 24/7 mental health crisis by 2021 (NHS England Digital n.d.-g). Typically, CRHT's gatekeep the inpatient beds within services and help to facilitate early discharge and reduce the length of hospital admissions (Royal College of Psychiatrists 2022).

Home treatment for crisis resolution should be:

- Available over 7 days a week.
- Provide home assessment, treatment, intervention and support offering an alternative to hospital admission.
- Provide support to the care coordination of community teams.
- Provide short-term interventions and managements of an individuals' care during periods of relapse.
- Continue until the crisis has been resolved.

Referral to CRHT's does vary across the country. However, as a minimum, referrals should be accepted from:

- Self-referrals/relatives/others.
- Ambulance/street triage/ED.
- GPs.
- Community mental health teams.
- CAMHS services.
- AMPH services.
- On call doctors.
- Outpatient clinics.
- Mental health assessment units.
- Liaison psychiatry services.
- Inpatient services.
- Section 136 suites.

Crisis Houses

They are typically smaller than inpatient mental health wards and normally offer no more than ten beds. They are more often located in normal residential streets. Crisis houses vary in the extent of medical cover provided and there is variation in the mental health professional staff cover. Whilst some crisis houses are offered by the NHS, many are offered by the voluntary sector. However, they are all highly integrated services and work closely with acute and crisis resolution teams (Sweeney et al. 2014). In 2023, just over 50% of Clinical Commission Groups had crisis house offerings. This compares to 65% having police street triage and 63% having crisis telephone line (Sweeney et al. 2014).

Primary Care/GP

Mental Health in Primary Care

Primary care is often the first point of contact for people who are experiencing a mental health problem (NHS England 2019). An average GP list of 2000 service users will have (at any one time):

- 352 service users with a common mental health problem.
- 8 with psychosis.
- 180 with drug or alcohol dependency.
- 352 with a sub-threshold common mental health problem.
- 120 with a sub-threshold psychosis.
- 176 with personality disorder.
- 125 with a long-term condition with a comorbid mental health problem.
- 100 with medically unexplained symptoms (RCGP 2017).

How well GPs are positioned to manage mental health is up for debate. A systematic review looking to GP's perspectives of suicide prevention in primary care found four main themes: challenges to managing suicidal behaviours; fragmented relationships with mental health services; personal attitudes of GPs regarding suicidal behaviour and identified needs to improve suicide prevention in primary care (Marshall et al. 2025).

Challenges to Managing Suicidal Behaviours

GPs described challenges when managing suicidal behaviours. GPs identified concerns with time constraints within a consultation, and there were also concerns about different service user populations.

Lack of Support from Mental Health Services

GPs described often feeling frustrated by secondary care services, and the lack of support in managing acutely ill service users. There were also concerns about the referral challenges into community mental health services.

Personal Attitudes of GPs Regarding Suicidal Behaviour

GPs described personal views towards challenges associated with suicide risk assessing and the use of screening tools. A common theme was that GPs find it difficult to predict suicide as presentations can be subtle and harder to detect than physical health complaints. GPs voiced disbelief of service users who had gone on to end their life after presenting as low risk (Marshall et al. 2025).

Equally, a recent NHS questionnaire sent to 5000 GPs in England found that hundreds of GPs in England have never refused to sign a service user off for mental health issues (BBC News 2026).

The current healthcare strategy is to return mental health nurses into multidisciplinary primary care teams. This is moving away from a secondary care model and moving towards multidisciplinary teams which are based around doctor's practices and service smaller populations (NHS England 2019). This strategy is part of the NHS Long Term Plan (NHS England 2019).

There are a number of benefits of integrating mental service in primary care:

Physical Health Needs

It means service users, specifically those who are older adults, can be treated for common mental health conditions at the same time as presenting with physical health needs. This moves much closer to the ideas of holistic and person-centred care.

Colocation

This allows sharing of knowledge between professionals and follows good practice to focus on holistic care (Lalani and Marshall 2022). Working physically together allows more opportunity for shared learning, as well as those more natural conversations between clinicians which help to share knowledge and experiences.

A study looking at a primary care mental health service looked into the effectiveness of the idea of mental health professionals working within integrated primary care services. They worked to the 'Stepped care' model of treatment for people with any mental health problems:

Step 1—This is the watchful waiting stage by the GP, who may also provide self-help information and continue to monitor patient's mental health over multiple appointments.

Step 2—Those in step 2 were treated by Psychological Wellbeing practitioners who support service users to use guided self-help programmes.

Step 3—Unresponsive service users with anxiety disorders and depression were referred to CBT therapists or counsellors who had post-graduate training in CBT, Counselling or Interpersonal Therapy. Service users with other diagnosis were treated by community mental health nurses in primary care.

Step 4—Service users who have complex needs involving multiple mental health professionals were 'stepped up' top psychiatrist-led community teams (Kenwright et al. 2024).

Results from this study demonstrated clinically significant pre to post-treatment effects in symptom reduction and functional improvement for service users treated by community mental health nurses for a range of mental health problems (Kenwright et al. 2024). They identified that the aids to integration were a single line of clinical management and governance; shared training across all roles; a shared IT system/electronic appointment diary. The barriers identified were around contract management structures, and different IT systems across primary and secondary care (Kenwright et al. 2024). It is important to consider how often you work alongside mental health clinicians as there is clear value in this, or whether there is opportunity for you to work in the same location as them more often.

NHS Talking Therapies

NHS Talking Therapies provide psychological therapy and intervention for adults in England who are struggling with anxiety disorders and/or depression. This service offers National Institute of Clinical Excellence (NICE) talking therapies that are tailored to service user's needs. Talking Therapies offer a range of different deliveries including face-to-face, remote, individual and group therapies.

NHS Talking Therapies was initially known as Improving access to Psychological Therapies (IAPT) and began in 2008. In 2023/24, 670,000 people received a course of treatment with further expansion planned for the coming 5 years (NHS England n.d.-d).

NHS Talking Therapies offer treatment for adults with the following common mental health problems:

- Agoraphobia.
- Body dysmorphic disorder.
- Depression.
- Generalised anxiety disorder.
- Health anxiety.
- Mixed depression and anxiety.
- Panic disorder.
- Post-traumatic stress disorder.
- Social anxiety disorder.
- Specific phobias (NHS England 2026).

Talking Therapies offer a range of NICE recommended therapies:

- Guided self-help based on cognitive behavioural therapy principles.
- Cognitive behavioural therapy.
- Interpersonal therapy.
- Couple therapy for depression or behavioural couple therapy.
- Dynamic interpersonal therapy.
- Counselling for depression.

- Mindfulness-based cognitive therapy.
- Trauma-focused cognitive behavioural therapy.
- Eye movement desensitisation and reprocessing (NHS England 2026).

Statistics from 2024 to 2025 suggested that Cognitive Behavioural Therapy and Guided Self Help (Book) accounted for 71.9% of all courses of therapy given. Of all the therapies, interpersonal psychotherapy had the highest rates of recovery and improvement (NHS Digital 2025).

Social Prescribing

Social prescribing is an important component of Universal Personalised Care (NHS England n.d.-c). Social prescribing involves connecting individuals to community groups and activities to support mental health and wellbeing (Aughterson et al. 2024). These are non-medical interventions to address wider determinants of health (Drinkwater et al. 2019). Evidence suggests that social prescribing can be used by all ages but can be particularly effective in those who have one or more long-term condition, who have support with low-level mental health issues, lonely or isolated, or have complex social needs which affect their wellbeing (NHS England n.d.-a)

Social prescribing recognises that people's health is determined by social, economic and environmental factors. It recognises that people need to be viewed in a holistic way (Gov.uk 2022).

What sorts of activities can be provided under social prescribing?

- Arts, culture, and heritage-based activities—such as music, art groups, and museum sessions.
- Physical activity.
- Education and welfare support sessions—this can include sessions such as employment support, financial advice, and fuel poverty support.
- Natural-based activities—such as gardening or nature walks (King's Fund 2026).

A model of social prescribing has been developed by NHS England in partnership with stakeholders and demonstrates the elements which need to be in place for effective social prescribing to happen. Please see the model, Fig. 1, of social prescribing below. (NHS England n.d.-c)

Did You Know?

New research suggests that parkrun is saving NHS England money in the treatment of key health conditions with 7 in 10 Britons also backing GPs to socially prescribe parkrun to service users. Data from Sports England suggests direct cost savings to NHS in the preventative treatment of depression (£13.8 million), type 2 diabetes

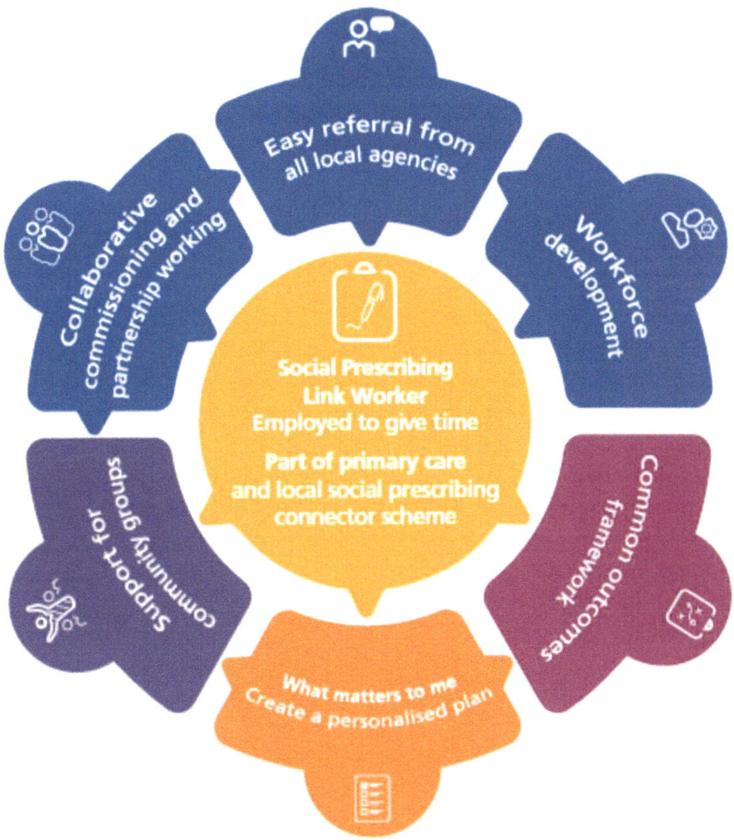

Easy referral from all local agencies
Workforce development
Common outcomes framework
What matters to me
Create a personalised plan
Support for community groups
Collaborative commissioning and partnership working
Social Prescribing Link Worker
Employed to give time
Part of primary care and local social prescribing connector scheme

Fig. 1 Standard model of social prescribing (NHS England Digital n.d.-c) (Published in https://www.england.nhs.uk/personalisedcare/social-prescribing/, under Open Government Licence v3.0)

(£13.5 million) and in reduced GP and hospital visits (£9.2 million) by people taking part with parkrun or the charity's parkrun practice social prescribing programme with the Royal College of GPs (parkrun UK 2026).

A national, longitudinal observational study looked at 1.2 million service users from 1736 GP practices in the Clinical Practice Research Datalink in England. The study aimed to assess longitudinal trends in social prescribing in England's primary care system. The findings of this study showed that 9.4 million GP consultations in England have involved social prescribing codes, and 5.5 million consultations have led to direct social prescribing referrals. About 60% of service users offered social prescribing were female, and 23% were from ethnic minority groups. The refusal of social prescribing referrals declined between 2019 and 2023. The referrals of social prescribing significantly exceeded targets which suggests there was broad acceptability of the scheme across medical practitioners and service users (Bu et al. 2025).

Community

One of the challenges of community mental health care is that people are often discharged out to the community with very little support. Equally, others who are waiting in the community are having long and frustrating waits to access care. Some people cannot access the care that they need because of tight, and very inflexible, referral and admission criteria (Health and Social Care Committee 2025)

A study was completed into the experience of staff in NHS and third sectors mental health care in England. These studies can often be useful to understand the perspectives and efficacy of mental health service provision in the community. The findings of this study suggest that community services are in crisis, with a focus on stabilisation of symptoms rather than rehabilitation. There was also a lack of provision, and services are stretched beyond coping point. There was an overall focus on crisis management and stabilisation, rather than overall recovery and approaches such as risk aversion which do not promote person-centred care. Finally, participants reported that there was evidence of situational unhappiness which does not require formal intervention and a lingering overreliance on the medical model. Participants also report inefficient pathways for people with complex mental health needs and often unsuitable pathways for individuals with complex needs. There was often a lack of mutual respect between sectors, which impacted barriers to collaboration. There was also evidence of clinical snobbery (Sambrook et al. 2025).

Community services vary by area and Trust, and this section will cover some of the most common that you may work with. However, services will vary slightly by name depending on region.

Community Mental Health Framework for Adults and Older Adults

The introduction of the Community Mental Health Framework, Fig. 2, was a huge structural shift in mental health and marked the end of the Care Programme Approach. The Care Programme Approach had been in use for almost 30 years, and one you may have seen in use within your own clinical practice (NHS England 2026).

This framework gives a foundation for the delivery of mental health care in their homes and communities. This was introduced as part of the NHS Long Term Plan. It provides a plan that offers a new community-based offering that includes access to psychological therapies, improved physical health care, employment support,

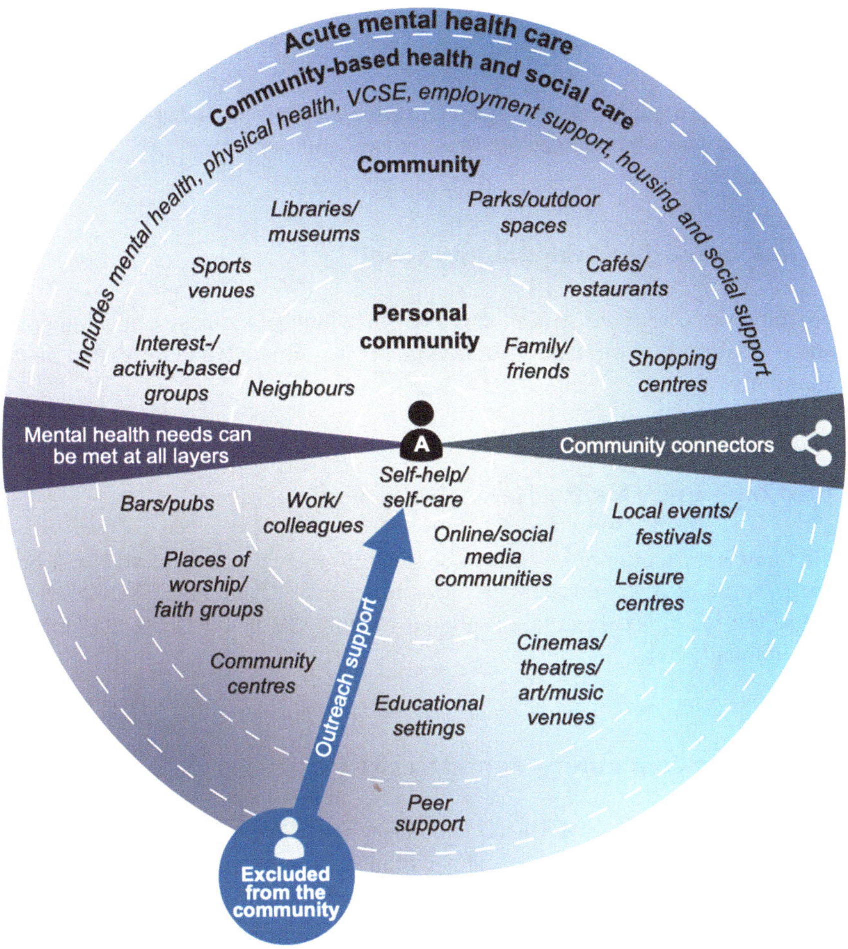

Fig. 2 Community Mental Health Framework. (Published in https://www.england.nhs.uk/publication/the-community-mental-health-framework-for-adults-and-older-adults/, under Open Government Licence v3.0)

personalised and trauma-informed care, medicines management and support for self-harm and coexisting substance use.

The key aims of the framework are the following:

1. Promote mental health and physical health and then also to prevent ill health.
2. Treat mental health problems effectively through evidence-based approaches, and using a collaborative approach.
3. Improve quality of life and involvement in communities.
4. Maximise continuity of care.
5. Work collaboratively across statutory and non-statutory commissioners and providers across health and care to address health inequalities and social determinants of mental ill health.

6. Build a model of care based on inclusivity (NHS England and NHS Improvement and National Collaborating Centre for Mental Health 2019).

This has been used under the Open Government License v.3.0.

The structure of this framework looks at five main sections:

Neighbourhood and Community Level

The framework sets out a new approach in which place-based and integrated mental health support, care and treatment are situated and provided in the community.

Core Community Mental Health Service

This framework that proposes a core community mental health service will bring together primary care services and secondary care Community Mental Health Teams (CMHT's). These are built around existing GP practices, neighbourhoods and community hubs.

Functions of Community Mental Health Provision

Key functions will be provided in the community and delivered from the Framework's place-based and integrated model. This will include services such as advocacy services, coordination and delivery of care, employment, education, volunteering and training services, and housing and social case services.

Mental Health Services for People with More Complex Needs

These services will be part of the same system of care and have close links with communities. However, these will provide capacity and expertise to deliver care to people with more complex needs. This includes services such as crisis and inpatient care. It also provides support and intensive and assertive support to communities such as rough sleepers, socially excluded people and people leaving the criminal justice service.

Accessing Care

In this framework, assessment is biopsychosocial and forms part of the integrated team approach to assessment. Assessment will be undertaken by different members of the core community mental health service at the point at which a person seeks access (NHS England 2019).

Lone Working

Reflective Questions
What is your long working policy in your workplace?
How confident do you feel in lone working?

An interesting study was done with Birmingham and Solihull Mental Health Foundation Trust's (BSMHFT) resident doctors. The aim of this was to improve the awareness and adherence to lone working policy amongst Resident doctors in inpatient and community settings and to standardise lone working processes across BSMHFT. Work was done to incorporate the lone work checklist into orientation checklists, lone working presentation at orientation, video on lone working and alarm use and clinical supervisee reminders. Results showed that there was an improvement in confidence when lone working and confidence in using alarms (Khan et al. 2025).

The examination of mental health environments illustrates where the system excels and where there is ongoing strain. There is evidence of significant policy development, such as Mental Health A + E and The Community Mental Health Framework. However, themes such as fragmentation, overstretched capacity and inconsistencies show how ongoing NHS structural issues can impact service user experience.

Social prescribing and renewed efforts in Primary Care have been shown to make real differences to service user care. These ideas alone have started to show that the NHS can look at mental health in a biopsychosocial sphere. They have highlighted the importance of collaboration, flexibility and person-centred care.

Design for Safety and Dignity

Reflective Questions
What do you think the positives and negatives are in the design of your workspace for clinicians and for service users?
Do you think that your environment promotes dignity for service users?

In mental health services, there has long been a tension between safety and dignity. Safety has often come at the cost of personal space, respect and dignity (Building Better Healthcare 2024). Mental health services are not alone with this, with private conversations still happening behind flimsy curtains and open waiting rooms in many other fields of health care.

However, it is still normal in some services to be asked to give in your personal items on admission, and in some parts of the world and the UK, wear poor quality hospital-issued clothing for protection (Building Better Healthcare 2024). For example, you may be asked to give in belts or shoelaces, phones, shavers or anything else felt 'risky' to have in your private space. In the first acute ward I worked in, the walls had not been plastered, and the painted breeze block was a light-yellow colour.

Doors within mental health services pose the biggest risk. About 51% of inpatient suicides involve a door, or the hardware around a door, and this is a significantly bigger risk than windows. About 91% of suicides occur in the service user's bedroom or bathroom—a place where privacy is clearly key but has the highest risks (National Confidential Inquiry into Suicide and Safety in Mental Health 2024).

CCTV and cameras are increasingly being used in a service user's room. In some cases, these cameras can also be used to track a service user's pulse and breathing (BBC 2025). The Lampard Inquiry has also raised significant concerns about the use of digital patient monitoring systems within patient rooms, specifically those which use infrared sensors and cameras to monitor service users alone in their bedrooms (BBC 2025).

An interesting study was completed in Australia around the redesign of a regional mental health unit. The aim of the study was to obtain user perspectives to inform the redesign of the mental health unit. Focus groups and interviews were undertaken during the process of planning for redesign. Three main themes were found within this study. Firstly, rooms should be designed to ensure and promote physical safety; purposeful planning to support interactions between users and systems will promote relational safety and optimising service integrity should promote procedural safety (Wilson et al. 2022).

Theme 1—Rooms Designed to Promote Physical Safety

- Adoption of therapeutic landscape in indoor and outdoor rooms which will accommodate diversity, acuity and rurality.
- An integrative architectural precinct should combine the main hospital with a mental health unit, which allows all-weather access.
- Bedrooms should be ensuite.
- Selection of materials and technologies should enable intensive treatment together with privacy and observability to minimise risks.
- These principles need to be balanced with aesthetics that promote recovery in the context of person-centred and trauma-informed care.

Theme 2—Purposeful Planning of Interactions

- Design should mitigate disruption, alleviate boredom and promote hospitality,
- Nursing stations should avoid a 'fishbowl' design.
- Promote wayfinding and easy navigation.
- Enhance relational security.

Theme 3—Optimising Service Integrity Will Promote Procedural Security

- Create a therapeutic environment.
- Design safe physical space to enable treatment, privacy and observability.
- Minimise, reduce and eliminate factors that perpetuate stigma around mental health.
- Apply the principles of person-centred and trauma-informed care to inform the design of the built environment.

Task

This is a task that I like to do with my second year adult nursing students. Thinking about everything learnt to date, please consider the following two questions:

How would you redesign your working environment to make it more suitable for those with mental health problems?
How would you design a mental health unit (choose the cohort that fits you best) to take into account all that you have learnt and reflected on so far?

It is interesting that with my last cohort, so many of the students chose to bring the 'outdoors in' and have big windows, indoor plants and bright, airy spaces including nature. If we think about many of the asylum buildings that we know—they had big windows and brought in light!

Key Learning Points

Mental health services work across a number of environments, some of which have been summarised in the chapter above. The environments that people seek care will influence the distress, risk and behaviours.

People will often access care in urgent health services, such as A + E, due to systems pressures and difficulties in understanding what services to manage. People may present to your service due to resource gap and not personal choice.

A + E and urgent care services are often distressing and overstimulating for those people in mental health crisis. It is important that you understand what you can do within your service to prioritise de-escalation, sensory awareness, and trauma-informed care.

Liaison psychiatry and mental health crisis services are an important aspect of mental health care, and in bridging the gap between mental health and physical health services. It is important you understand how these services work within your service, and how you can access them.

Social prescribing is an important tool for holistic and person-centred care. We should all understand what local services may support our service users.

Conclusion

Mental health care happens everywhere. Much of our mental health care may happen in complex and overstretched environments. As discussed within the chapter, environments such as A + E departments, primary care and acute inpatient units offer unique benefits and challenges to how people access care.

A + E services remain a key access point for many in crisis, and it is often an overstimulating and emotionally challenging environment for those people in mental health distress. Unpredictability, overcrowding and long waits may contribute to increased agitation and poorer outcomes for service users who present there. However, there has been increased work on looking at alternatives for this service user group. Mental health A + Es or MUHAC units offer a good alternative to people within this group, although fragmentation and separation of physical and mental health remain concerns across some groups.

Primary care remains the most common entry point for mental health concerns. However, GPs face challenges with time, knowledge and understanding. Equally, community services are going through a period of change as the Community Mental Health Framework continues to bed in. Community-based approaches have the potential to provide more holistic and recovery-focused support, but variations in funding, staffing, and accessibility continue to create inequalities in care provision across different regions and populations.

This chapter discusses the importance that environments play in shaping mental health service delivery and service user outcomes. By understanding the pressures, opportunities, and limitations of the environments discussed in this chapter, we can all advocate to deliver better, more knowledgeable, person-centred care. It is also important that practitioners remain aware of how environments influence not only service users, but also staff wellbeing, decision-making and therapeutic relationships. Safe, compassionate and recovery-focused environments can significantly improve engagement, trust and outcomes for those accessing mental health support. As healthcare systems continue to evolve, practitioners must continue reflecting on how services can become more accessible, integrated and responsive to the diverse needs of the populations they serve.

References

Aughterson H, Fancourt D, Chatterjee H, Burton A (2024) Social prescribing for individuals with mental health problems: an ethnographic study exploring the mechanisms of action through which community groups support psychosocial well-being. Wellcome Open Res 19(9):149. https://doi.org/10.12688/wellcomeopenres.20981.1. PMID: 38952567; PMCID: PMC11216282. Accessed 3 Apr 2026

Austin E, Cheek C, Richardson L, Testa L, Dominello A, Long JC, Carrigan A, Ellis LA, Norman A, Murphy M, Smith K, Gillies D, Clay-Williams R (2024) Improving emergency department care for adults presenting with mental illness: a systematic review of strategies and their impact on outcomes, experience, and performance. Front Psychiatry 15:1368129. https://doi.org/10.3389/fpsyt.2024.1368129. Accessed 15 Apr 2026

BBC News (2025) Lampard inquiry: 'grave concerns' about Oxevision monitoring system. BBC News. [Online] 14 Oct. Available at: https://www.bbc.co.uk/news/articles/cvgk399m70lo. Accessed 30 Mar 2026

BBC News (2026) Hundreds of GPs tell BBC they have never refused a sick note over mental health concerns. BBC News. [Online] 12 Mar. Available at: https://www.bbc.co.uk/news/articles/c20lew24kngo. Accessed 30 Mar 2026

Bu F, Burton A, Launders N, Taylor A, Richards-Belle A, Tierney S (2025) National roll-out of social prescribing in England's primary care system: a longitudinal observational study using Clinical Practice Research Datalink data. Lancet 10(11):E903–E911

Buchanan M (2024) Mental health and A&E: finding a path forward. NHS Confederation, 12 December. Available at: https://www.nhsconfed.org/news/mental-health-and-ae-finding-path-forward. Accessed 1 Jan 2026

Building Better Healthcare (2024) Made for living: the future of mental health. Available at: https://buildingbetterhealthcare.com/made-for-living-the-future-of-mental-health. Accessed: 6 Mar 2026

Care Quality Commission (2019) Shared sleeping arrangements on mental health wards (dormitories). Available at: https://www.cqc.org.uk/sites/default/files/Brief_guide_Shared_sleeping_arrangements_on_mental_health_wards_dormitories.pdf. Accessed 30 Mar 2026

Drinkwater, C., Wildman, J. Moffatt, S. (2019) Social prescribing. BMJ, 364, 11285. Available at: https://research.ncl.ac.uk/media/sites/researchwebsites/nuspemedia/Drinkwater%20et%20al%202019.pdf. Accessed 6 Feb 2026

Edge Health (2025) MHUAC evaluation—final report 29/03/23. Available at: https://www.edgehealth.co.uk/wp-content/uploads/2025/07/FINAL_MHUAC_Evaluation_290323.pdf. Accessed 30 Mar 2026

Evans-Lacko SE, Jarrett M, McCrone P, Thornicroft G. (2018) Clinical pathways in psychiatry. Br J Psychiatry 193(1):4–5. Available at: https://doi.org/10.1192/bjp.bp.107.048926. Accessed 12 Jan 2026

Gilburt H (2025) NHS reliant on beds in independent sector for mental health care. The King's Fund. Available at: https://www.kingsfund.org.uk/insight-and-analysis/long-reads/nhs-reliant-beds-independent-sector-mental-health-care. Accessed 3 Jan 2026

Gilburt H, Mallorie S (2024) Mental health 360: acute mental health care for adults. The King's Fund. Available at: https://www.kingsfund.org.uk/insight-and-analysis/long-reads/mental-health-360-acute-mental-health-care-adults. Accessed 3 Apr 2026

Health and Social Care Committee (2025) Community mental health services. Fourth Report of Session 2024–26. HC 566. London: House of Commons. Available at: https://committees.parliament.uk/publications/50484/documents/274145/default/. Accessed 1 June 2026

Kenwright M, Fairclough P, McDonald J, Pickford L (2024) Effectiveness of community mental health nurses in an integrated primary care service: an observational cohort study. Int J Nurs Stud Adv 6:100182. https://doi.org/10.1016/j.ijnsa.2024.100182. Accessed 18 July 2026

Khan T, Cheema K, Htwe Y, Liu H, Asim A (2025) 'Improving lone work practice within a mental health trust: a quality improvement project. BJPsych Open 11(Suppl. 1):S140. Available at: https://doi.org/10.1192/bjo.2025.10384. Accessed 3 Apr 2026.

King's Fund (2026) Social prescribing. Available at: https://www.kingsfund.org.uk/insight-and-analysis/long-reads/social-prescribing. Accessed 30 Mar 2026

LaingBuisson (2024) Independent sector mental health hospitals market valued at £2.36bn. Available at: https://www.laingbuisson.com/press-releases/independent-sector-mental-health-hospitals-market-valued-at-record-2-36-billion/. Accessed 30 Mar 2026

Lalani M, Marshall M (2022) Co-location, an enabler for service integration? Lessons from an evaluation of integrated community care teams in East London. Health Soc Care Community 30(2):e388–e396. Available at: https://doi.org/10.1111/hsc.13211. Accessed 3 Apr 2026

Lee K, Jang K, Kim H, Bae G, Jang CS, Shin JH (2023) Factors affecting the length of stay in the emergency department in psychiatric emergency patients in the COVID-19 pandemic context. Inquiry: A Journal of Medical Care Organization, Provision and Financing 60:469580231167529. https://doi.org/10.1177/00469580231167529. Accessed 3 Apr 2026

Lloyd-Evans B, Johnson S (2019) Community alternatives to inpatient admissions in psychiatry. World Psychiatry, 18:31-32. https://doi.org/10.1002/wps.20587. Accessed 19 July 2026

Marshall J, Oliver P, Hulin J, Huddy V, Mitchell C (2025) General practitioners perspectives regarding suicide prevention: a systematic scoping review. BJGP Open 10(1). BJGPO.2024.0225. Available at: https://doi.org/10.3399/BJGPO.2024.0225. Accessed 12 Feb 2026

Mason S, Marincowitz C, Guthrie E (2025) Urgent care for mental health in the NHS', BMJ, 390, r1782. Available at: https://doi.org/10.1136/bmj.r1782. Accessed 2 Apr 2026

National Confidential Inquiry into Suicide and Safety in Mental Health (2024) Annual report 2024: UK patient and general population data 2011–2021. Manchester: The University of Manchester. Available at: https://sites.manchester.ac.uk/ncish/reports/annual-report-2024/. Accessed 12 Dec 2025

NHS Digital (2025) NHS Talking Therapies—therapy-based outcomes 2024–25. Available at: https://digital.nhs.uk/data-and-information/publications/statistical/nhs-talking-therapies-for-anxiety-and-depression-annual-reports/2024-25/therapy-based-outcomes. Accessed 30 Mar 2026

NHS England (2014) NHS England welcomes Crisis Care Concordat. 18 February. Available at: https://www.england.nhs.uk/2014/02/crisis-care-con/. Accessed 3 Apr 2026

NHS England (2019) Lord Carter's review into unwarranted variations in mental health and community health services. Available at: https://www.england.nhs.uk/publication/lord-carters-review-into-unwarranted-variations-in-mental-health-and-community-health-services/. Accessed 30 Mar 2026

NHS England (2025) New ambulances and faster emergency care for patients next winter. Available at: https://www.england.nhs.uk/2025/06/new-ambulances-and-faster-emergency-care-for-patients-next-winter/. Accessed 30 Mar 2026

NHS England (2026) Mental health personalised care framework: the modern care programme approach https://www.england.nhs.uk/long-read/mental-health-personalised-care-framework-the-modern-care-programme-approach/. Accessed 18 July 2026

NHS England Digital (n.d) Hospital bed types. Available at: https://digital.nhs.uk/data-and-information/data-collections-and-data-sets/data-collections/assuring-transformation/hospital-bed-types. Accessed 20 Feb 2026

NHS England (n.d.-a) Mental health and A&E: finding a path forward. Available at: https://www.nhsconfed.org/news/mental-health-and-ae-finding-path-forward. Accessed 30 Mar 2026

NHS England (n.d.-c) Personalised care: social prescribing. Available at: https://www.england.nhs.uk/personalisedcare/social-prescribing/. Accessed 30 Mar 2026

NHS England (n.d.-d) NHS Talking Therapies. Available at: https://www.england.nhs.uk/mental-health/adults/nhs-talking-therapies/. Accessed 30 Mar 2026

NHS England (n.d.-g) Crisis and acute mental health services Available at: https://www.england.nhs.uk/mental-health/adults/crisis-and-acute-care/. Accessed 20 March 2026

NHS England and NHS Improvement and National Collaborating Centre for Mental Health (2019) The Community Mental Health Framework for Adults and Older Adults. London: NHS England. Available at: https://www.england.nhs.uk/wpcontent/uploads/2019/09/community-mental-health-framework-for-adults-and-older-adults.pdf. Accessed 9 Jan 2026

Raja U, Misra A, Kar N (2024) Change in risk status of psychiatric patients admitted to Crisis and Home Treatment Team: an evaluation in the UK. European Psychiatry 67(Suppl 1), S571. https://doi.org/10.1192/j.eurpsy.2024.1188. Accessed 12 Feb 2026

RCGP (2017) Mental health in primary care. Available at: https://www.rcgp.org.uk/representing-you/policy-areas/mental-health-in-primary-care. Accessed 30 Mar 2026

Royal College of Psychiatrists (2022) Practice guidelines for crisis line response and Crisis Resolution and Home Treatment Teams (CRHTTs). London: Royal College of Psychiatrists. Available at: https://www.rcpsych.ac.uk/docs/default-source/improving-care/ccqi/quality-networks/htas/practice-guidelines-for-crisis-line-response-and-crhtt's-2022.pdf. Accessed 3 Apr 2026

Royal College of Psychiatrists (2025) RCPsych responds to plans to open mental health A&E centres across England. Available at: https://www.rcpsych.ac.uk/news-and-features/latest-news/detail/2025/05/29/rcpsych-responds-to-plans-to-open-mental-health-a-e-centres-across-england. Accessed 30 Mar 2026

Parkrun UK (2026) New data shows parkrun's savings to NHS England. 26 March. Available at: https://blog.parkrun.com/uk/2026/03/26/new-data-shows-parkruns-savings-to-nhs-england/ Accessed: 10 May 2026

Sambrook L, McIntyre JC, Nathan R, Tait J, Ashley-Mudie P, Humphreys M, Wilson P, Saini P (2025) 'A community in crisis': staff qualitative experiences of NHS and third sector mental healthcare in England. BJPsych Open 11(5):e210. https://doi.org/10.1192/bjo.2025.10826

Sampson EL, Wright J, Dove J, Mukadam N, Shetty H (2022) Psychiatric liaison service referral patterns during the UK COVID-19 pandemic: an observational study. Eur J Psychiatry 36(1):35–42. Available at: https://doi.org/10.1016/j.ejpsy.2021.05.003. Accessed 3 Apr 2026

Sweeney A, Fahmy S, Nolan F, Morant N, Fox Z, Lloyd-Evans B, Osborn D, Burgess E, Gilburt H, McCabe R, Slade M, Johnson S (2014) The relationship between therapeutic alliance and service user satisfaction in mental health inpatient wards and crisis house alternatives: a cross-sectional study. PLoS One 9(7):e100153. https://doi.org/10.1371/journal.pone.0100153. Erratum in: PLoS One 9(10):e110097. PMID: 25010773; PMCID: PMC4091866. Accessed 3 Apr 2026

Taylor B (2026) The changing terrain of mental health in A&E: specialised care or the same old bottlenecks? QualityWatch: Nuffield Trust and Health Foundation

The Health Foundation (n.d.) Safer care pathways in mental health services. Available at: https://www.health.org.uk/improvement-projects/safer-care-pathways-in-mental-health-services. Accessed 8 Apr 2026

Whittle C (2007) Introduction to ICPs. National Health Service. Available at: http://www.library.nhs.uk/pathways/ViewResource.aspx?resID=259106&tabID=290&catID=12584. Accessed 30 Mar 2026

Wilson RL, Hutton A, Foureur M (2022) Promoting mental health recovery by design: physical, procedural, and relational security in the context of the mental health built environment. Int J Ment Health Nurs 32(1):147–161. https://doi.org/10.1111/inm.13070

Pharmacology and Therapeutic Treatments

Assets

The major classes of drugs in mental health are the following:

1. Anxiolytics (hypnotics).
2. Antipsychotics.
3. Antidepressants.
4. Antimanics.
5. Stimulants.
6. Anticonvulsants.
7. Sedatives.

The routes of drug administration can be seen in Table 1 (Kim and De Jesus 2023; Thompson and DiMartini 1999).

Antidepressants

The main neurotransmitters thought to be involved in depression are the monoamines—serotonin and noradrenaline (Blows 2022).

Tricyclic Antidepressants

These are medications named after the three-ringer (tri-cyclic) nature (or the dibenzoazepine structure) (Blows 2022). They work by blocking the uptake of the neurotransmitters, serotonin and noradrenaline into the presynaptic bulb. This leads

R. Bage, *Mental Health Skills for Adult Nurses & Non-Specialist Healthcare Workers*, https://doi.org/10.1007/978-3-032-32835-9_9

Table 1 Routes of drug administration

Route of administration	Details	Strengths	Weaknesses
Oral	This is by mouth and is a convenient method for service users who can ingest and tolerate oral medication. Some medications with short half-lives are administered orally as time-released or sustained release.	Easy to administer Widespread acceptability by service users—does not make them feel 'different'. Cheap and easy	Variable absorption rates Can have some degradation of drugs before reaching the site or absorption Some compounds cannot effectively traverse the intestinal epithelial membrane cells to reach blood Potential irritation of mucous lining of the gastrointestinal tract Potential inactivation of the drugs in liver on the way to the systemic circulation
Intravenous	Widely used for general anaesthesia, sedating agitating service users and relieving symptoms of anxiety	Good distribution by avoidance of first-pass metabolism	Some medications do not come in intravenous forms, e.g. antidepressants In many cases, these are not licensed for mental health administration
Intramuscular	This is a route used often in mental health practice due to fast absorption and increased bioavailability	Used regularly for rapid tranquilisation and depot antipsychotics	Cannot be used for service users with reduced muscle perfusion Difficult to daily injections of some drugs as may cause irritation, necrosis, or abscesses
Subcutaneous	Medication is injected into the fatty tissue beneath the skin, commonly in the abdomen, thigh or upper arm. Used for insulin, heparin and some biologic medications.	Slower absorption. Suitable for self-administration. Useful for medications destroyed in the gastrointestinal tract.	Requires needles and injections May cause pain Can cause infection at injection site Limited volume can be administered.

(continued)

Table 1 (continued)

Route of administration	Details	Strengths	Weaknesses
Rectal	This is used mainly by service users with gastrointestinal mobility problems—e.g. dysphagia The rectal route may also be used in service users who may be end of life	A large amount of drug can be administered Those drugs impacted by acidic nature of stomach can be administered effectively Safe administration for infants and the elderly Can be useful in emergency situations, such as infants having seizures Bypasses hepatic metabolism	Some drugs (e.g. antibiotics) are unsuitable for rectal administration as they are not easily absorbed May cause rectal irritation and proctitis—this can lead to ulceration and bleeding
Inhalation	Medication is breathed into the lungs Often used for inhalers/nebulisers	Very effective in treatment for respiratory conditions e.g. asthma or COPD Rapid onset of action Medication delivered directly to lugs	Technique dependent—service users may struggle to use inhalers correctly Can cause oral infections if mouth not rinsed
Topical	Medication is applied directly to the skin or mucous membranes as creams, ointments, gels or patches. Often used for skin conditions or local pain relief.	Not invasive Targeted local effect Reduced systemic side effects Convenient for service users	Can cause skin irritation Slower onset for some medication
Sublingual	These are for medications with high first-pass metabolism that needs to avoid the liver.	Rapid absorption due to mucosal network of systemic veins and lymphatics Tablet can be removed if required Avoids first-pass hepatic metabolism Useful for those with swallowing difficulties Low risk of infection Convenience	Must be kept in the buccal cavity and neither chewed nor swallowed Excessive salivation may cause quick dissolution and absorption of the tablet Service users may find it unpalatable

serotonin and noradrenaline to accumulate in the synaptic cleft. Medications within this category include doxepin, clomipramine, dosulepin and nortriptyline (Blows 2022).

The main challenge with this group of medications is the therapeutic delay. This means that these medications may not start making a difference for up to 6 weeks. The reason for this delay is thought to be related to the time it takes to down-regulate the receptors or to improve receptor sensitivity (Blows 2022). This causes challenges within mental health due to the risk of suicide because a patient might acquire more energy, which may lead to having more energy to undertake the act of suicide (Blows 2022).

The adverse effects of tricyclic medication have been highlighted in the Table 2 (NICE 2025).

Table 2 Adverse effects of tricyclic medication

Adverse effect	Very common side effects	Common	Less common
Cardiac	Tachycardia	Bundle branch block QT interval prolongation	Palpitations Arrhythmias AV block Hypertension Myocardial infarction Sudden cardiac death
Visual	Accommodation disorder	Mydriasis	Blurred Vision
Gastrointestinal			Dry mouth Appetite (reduced) Altered taste Constipation Nausea Diarrhoea Vomiting Abdominal pain Paralytic ileus Changes to weight
Central nervous system			Somnolence Tremor Dizziness Reduced concentration Confusion Headache Drowsiness Speech changes/Disorders Peripheral neuropathy Seizure Sleep disorders Tinnitus

(continued)

Table 2 (continued)

Adverse effect	Very common side effects	Common	Less common
Psychiatric	Aggression		Confusion Anxiety Agitation Delirium Hallucinations Suicidal behaviours
Skin			Skin reactions Alopecia Facial oedema Photosensitivity reactions
Other			Bone marrow depression Gynaecomastia Hyperhidrosis Hyponatraemia Neuroleptic malignant syndrome Sexual dysfunction Thrombocytopenia Urinary disorders

There are also several known drug interactions with tricyclic antidepressants which include:

- Clonidine—The antihypertensive effects may be reduced by tricyclic antidepressants. Please be cautious about those on clonidine.
- Lithium—Lithium is a medication used frequently as a mood stabiliser, and you will see discussed further down in this chapter. Concurrent use with a tricyclic antidepressant may cause neurotoxicity, serotonin syndrome or neuroleptic malignant syndrome (Health Education England, n.d.-a). Both drugs are linked QT interval prolongation or torsade's de pointes.
- Monoamine oxidase inhibitors (MAOIs)—Concurrent use is contraindicated due to risks of serotonin syndrome or similar.
- Other sedative drugs (alcohol, barbiturates and benzodiazepines)—TCAs are sedating and coadministration with other sedating drugs may have a synergistic effect.
- Phenothiazines—Concentrations of both drugs may be increased, increasing the risk of tardive dyskinesia and antimuscarinic adverse effects. In addition, risk of QT interval prolongation if both drugs are taken concomitantly.
- Selective serotonin reuptake inhibitors (SSRIs) and serotonin noradrenaline reuptake inhibitors (SNRIs)—TCA concentrations may be increased leading to adverse effects. SSRIs and SNRIs particularly are also associated with QT interval prolongation, possibly increasing the risk of arrhythmias if taken with a TCA.
- Tramadol—May increase the risk of serotonin syndrome. You will need to check whether any service user is on tramadol.
- Warfarin—TCAs may affect the prothrombin time. You will need to check whether any service user is on warfarin (NICE 2025).

What Is Serotonin Syndrome?

Serotonin syndrome occurs when there is too much accumulation of serotonin neurotransmitter in the body. The common symptoms are included in Fig. 1 (Health Education England n.d.-b; Mwebe 2021).

This likelihood of serotonin syndrome occurring is more likely if treated on a selective serotonin reuptake inhibitor (SSRI) and a MAOI. It is therefore advised to have a drug-free window before changing between a SSRI and a MAOI (between 2 and 5 weeks) (Mwebe 2021). Other medications implicated in serotonin syndrome include:

- Antidepressants, St John's wort, lithium.
- Tramadol, pethidine, fentanyl.
- Ondansetron, metoclopramide.
- Cocaine, MDMA, amphetamines, LSD (Health Education England n.d.-b).

Ward-based management of serotonin syndrome should include:

- Organise medical review.
- All medications should be reviewed.
- Fluids should be given for dehydration.
- Patient should be cooled down.
- Physical observations should be taken including heart rate, blood pressure, temperature, respiratory rate (Health Education England n.d.-b).

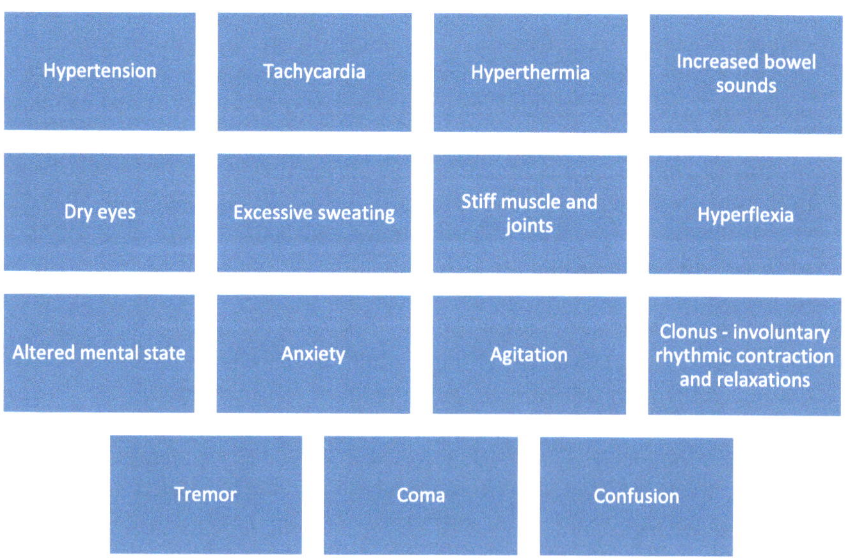

Fig. 1 Signs and symptoms of serotonin syndrome

Selective Serotonin Reuptake Inhibitors (SSRI)

SSRIs are the most commonly prescribed antidepressants for depression worldwide (Johnson et al. 2022). However, there is evidence to suggest that doses of SSRI medication have increased (Johnson et al. 2022). These drugs inhibit the reuptake of serotonin and increase the quantity of serotonin in the cleft. SSRI medications are said to have fewer side effects. They are also safer regards suicide risk, with tricyclic medication particularly risky in overdoses due to cardiac effects (Blows 2010). The SSRI medication also has fewer antimuscarinic side effects, and the known adverse effects are included in Table 3 (NICE 2022). Common side effects are nausea, vomiting, dizziness, fatigue and headaches. Some of these are more common in the first few weeks of taking the medication (Blows 2010).

Table 3 Adverse effects of SSRI medication

Adverse effect	Very common side effects	Common	Less common	Uncommon
Cardiac		Palpitations	QT interval prolongation Torsade de pointes (citalopram or escitalopram)	Tachycardia
Gastrointestinal			Reduced appetite Diarrhoea Nausea (dose-related) Dry mouth Abdominal pain Constipation Vomiting Altered taste Weight changes	Hepatitis
Central nervous system			Headache Dizziness Drowsiness Tinnitus Paraesthesia Tremor Sleep disorder Visual Impairment	Convulsions Movement disorders Serotonin syndrome
Psychiatric	Insomnia Anxiety		Agitation Confusion Reduced concentration Memory loss Depersonalisation	Mania

(continued)

Table 3 (continued)

Adverse effect	Very common side effects	Common	Less common	Uncommon
Skin	Hyperhidrosis		Rash Alopecia Puritius Photosensitive	Urticaria
Other			Haemorrhage Menstrual cycle irregularities Myalgia Sexual dysfunction Urinary disorders	Hyponatraemia Syndrome of inappropriate anti-diuretic hormone secretion Thrombocytopenia Leukopenia (Paroxetine only)

SSRIs should not be prescribed to:

- In a manic phase of a bipolar disorder.
- With poorly controlled epilepsy.
- With existing QT interval prolongation, or congenital long QT syndrome (citalopram and escitalopram).
- Concurrent use of drugs known to prolong the QT interval (citalopram and escitalopram).
- With severe hepatic impairment (sertraline).

There are also several known drug interactions with SSRI antidepressants which include:

- Antiepileptics—SSRIs can reduce the seizure threshold and make somebody more at risk of seizures. Please be aware of anyone who has a history of seizures when on SSRI medication and make sure they are also aware of the risks.
- Antidiabetic drugs—SSRIs can affect diabetic control. Monitor blood glucose when starting or stopping an SSRI.
- Aspirin, NSAIDs, anticoagulants, and antiplatelets—Increased risk of bleeding if taken concomitantly with SSRIs. Consider additional INR monitoring with warfarin.
- Carbamazepine—Levels of sertraline may be reduced.
- Cocaine—Possibly an increased risk of bleeding with citalopram. Clinicians should enquire about illicit drug use before prescribing SSRIs and make sure this is well documented.
- Grapefruit juice—Levels of sertraline may be modestly increased.
- HIV protease inhibitors (e.g. lopinavir, atazanavir)—Efficacy of SSRIs may be reduced. Monitor and adjust dose of SSRI if required.
- Lithium—Concurrent use with SSRI may cause serotonin syndrome or neuroleptic malignant syndrome. In addition, lithium has been associated with QT prolongation and concomitant use may increase this risk. Monitor for adverse effects.

- Monoamine oxidase inhibitors (MAOIs)—Concurrent use is contraindicated. Fatal reactions may occur (serotonin syndrome or neuroleptic malignant syndrome).
- SNRIs (venlafaxine, duloxetine)—Increased risk of serotonin syndrome or neuroleptic malignant syndrome when given concomitantly with an SSRI. Monitor for symptoms such as fever, tremor, diarrhoea, and agitation.
- Venlafaxine may also increase the risk of QT interval prolongation if taken concomitantly with an SSRI. It may be appropriate to consider ECG monitoring in this case.
- Other sedative drugs (alcohol, barbiturates, benzodiazepines)—SSRIs are sedating and coadministration with other sedating drugs may have a synergistic effect. Please ensure service users are aware of risks regards driving.
- Other drugs, which if taken with SSRIs may increase the risk of serotonin syndrome or neuroleptic malignant syndrome, include opioids, St John's wort (avoid concurrent use), triptans and vortioxetine. Please ensure that you are asking service users about St John's Wart as this is often used over the counter.
- QT interval prolongation—Some SSRIs are associated with QT interval prolongation and torsade de pointes. Concurrent use with other drugs that prolong the QT interval drugs may increase the risk. These include antiarrhythmics (amiodarone, dronedarone and quinidine); antipsychotics (phenothiazine derivatives, pimozide, haloperidol); tricyclic antidepressants (TCAs, clomipramine and imipramine); and sildenafil.
- Hyponatraemia—Increased risk if concurrent use with other drugs known to be associated with hyponatraemia (e.g. diuretics, NSAIDs, antipsychotics, carbamazepine, calcium channel blockers, angiotensin-converting enzyme [ACE] inhibitors and laxatives) (NICE 2025).

SSRIs are typically better tolerated by older service users and are recommended as a first-line treatment for all age groups as they are tolerated better than other antidepressant medications. SSRIs are widely prescribed in primary care services and are considered as an effective, safe and tolerable treatment. However, some children and younger adults are more likely to have suicidal thoughts when taking an SSRI, and this group should be monitored regularly (Mwebe 2021).

Serotonin and Noradrenaline Reuptake Inhibitors (SNRIs)

These drugs are similar to the tricyclic drugs as they block to reuptake of serotonin and noradrenaline. They have fewer side effects and a shorter therapeutic delay than the tricyclic medication, making them a safer choice (Blows 2010). The most common medication you may see within this group is venlafaxine.

Common side effects are the following:

- Nausea.
- Dizziness.
- Dry mouth.
- Sweating.
- Headaches.
- Male sexual dysfunction.
- Increased or irregular menstrual bleeding.
- Loss of appetite.
- Palpitations.
- Pins and needles.
- Raised blood pressure.
- Sight problems.
- Sleepiness (Blows 2010; Mwebe 2021).

SNRI medication should not be prescribed to those with:

- Uncontrolled hypertension.
- Hepatic impairment—duloxetine only.
- Severe renal impairment—duloxetine only.

SNRI should only be prescribed cautiously with:

- A history of bleed disorders.
- Susceptibility to angle-closure glaucoma—duloxetine only.
- Renal impairment—venlafaxine only.
- Hepatic impairment—venlafaxine only.
- Diabetes mellitus—blood sugar control can be affected by SNRI medication.
- Hypertension.
- Conditions which link to high risk of cardiac arrhythmia.
- Cardia disease (blood pressure monitoring is required).
- A history of family history of mania or bipolar disorder.
- Epilepsy (Joint Formulary Committee 2026d).

Venlafaxine is a medication with a very short half-life. This means that some people have problems when discontinuing the medication. This can include symptoms such as agitation, anxiety, depersonalisation, dizziness and nausea. It is recommended that the dose of venlafaxine is reduced slowly over a number of weeks to avoid these (Mwebe 2021).

There are also several drug interactions with use of serotonin noradrenaline reuptake inhibitors (SNRIs):

- Antifungals (fluconazole, itraconazole and ketoconazole)—Plasma concentration of venlafaxine increased. Manufacturer advises that concomitant use with fluconazole should only be undertaken with caution; for other antifungals monitor for adverse effects and adjust venlafaxine dose if necessary.

- Aspirin, NSAIDs, anticoagulants, and antiplatelets—Increased risk of bleeding if taken concurrently with SNRI. Consider additional INR monitoring if taking warfarin.
- Bupropion—Plasma concentration of SNRI increased. Monitor for adverse effects and adjust SNRI dose if necessary.
- Carvedilol, metoprolol—Levels may be increased by duloxetine. Monitor blood pressure.
- Ciprofloxacin—Avoid concomitant use (metabolism of duloxetine is inhibited by ciprofloxacin).
- Clarithromycin, erythromycin—Levels of venlafaxine may be increased. Possible increased risk of QT interval prolongation.
- Diltiazem, verapamil—Plasma concentration of venlafaxine may be increased. Monitor for adverse effects and adjust venlafaxine dose if necessary.
- HIV protease inhibitors (e.g. ritonavir, lopinavir and atazanavir): Levels of venlafaxine may be increased. Monitor for adverse effects and adjust dose of venlafaxine if necessary.
- Lithium—Concurrent use with SNRI may cause serotonin syndrome. In addition, lithium has been associated with QT interval prolongation. Monitor for adverse effects.
- Monoamine oxidase inhibitors (MAOIs)—Concurrent use is contraindicated. Fatal reactions may occur (serotonin syndrome).
- SSRIs (paroxetine, sertraline)—Increased risk of serotonin syndrome when given concurrently with an SNRI. Monitor for symptoms (such as fever, tremors, diarrhoea and agitation).
- Venlafaxine may also increase the risk of QT interval prolongation if taken concurrently with an SSRI. Consider ECG monitoring.
- Other sedative drugs (alcohol, barbiturates, and benzodiazepines)—SSRIs are sedating and coadministration with other sedating drugs may have a synergistic effect.
- Other drugs which if taken with an SNRI may increase the risk of serotonin syndrome include mirtazapine, opioids, St John's wort (avoid concurrent use), triptans and vortioxetine.
- QT interval prolongation—Possible increased risk of QT interval prolongation if venlafaxine is taken with other drugs known to cause QT interval prolongation, including antiarrhythmics (amiodarone, dronedarone and quinidine); antipsychotics (phenothiazine derivatives, pimozide and haloperidol); tricyclic antidepressants (TCAs, clomipramine and imipramine); sildenafil (Joint Formulary Committee 2026d; NICE 2025).

Monoamine Oxidase Inhibitors (MAOI)

The monoamine oxidase inhibitors block the enzyme monoamine oxidase. This is an enzyme on the outer membrane of mitochondria in the presynaptic bulb, and particularly involved in the dopaminergic, adrenergic and serotonergic pathways. This enzyme inactivates the neurotransmitter after its work in the presynaptic cleft and has been taken back to the bulb. When blocked, the neurotransmitter cannot be reduced for excretion and remains in the synapse. This leads to the transmitter levels rising in the bulb and cleft (Blows 2010).

There are two forms of MAO—MAO-A and MAO-B, although the brain has mostly MAO-B (Blows 2010). MAO-A mainly breaks down serotonin and noradrenaline, and MAO-B breaks down dopamine (Mwebe 2021). The MAOIs that are used to treat service users with depression are selective inhibitors of MAO-A (e.g. moclobemide) or non-selective MAOIs (e.g. isocarboxazid) (Mwebe 2021).

MAOI's come with a number of dietary restrictions. The MAO enzyme breaks down an excess of noradrenaline and tyramine, but when MAOI drugs are given, they interact with the metabolism of noradrenaline and tyramine. Excess of these two neurotransmitters can cause a dangerous increase in blood pressure and can cause a hypertensive crisis, stroke and death. However, there is lots of misinformation around dietary changes.

Overdosing on a MAOI can be fatal. Symptoms include drowsiness, dizziness, irritability, agitation, severe headaches, hallucinations, trismus, convulsions, rapid and irregular pulse, precordial pain, vascular collapse, respiratory depression and coma (Mwebe 2021).

Aminoketone (Bupropion)

This is a type of antidepressant but also acts as a stimulant. You may see it frequently used in smoking cessation. It is a noradrenaline and dopamine inhibitor and increases both of these chemicals within the brain. It reacts quicker than the tricyclic medication, typically around 4 weeks. It is also known to be associated with weight loss and should not be used in service users who have previously experienced an eating disorder. In the UK, this is not licensed for the treatment of severe depression, but you may see this used outside the terms of its license (Mwebe 2021).

Anxiolytics

Non-Benzodiazepine Hypnotics

'Z-drugs' include zopiclone, zolpidem, zaleplon and eszopiclone, and these work as benzodiazepine receptor agonists. They act as GABA agonists and increase the inhibitory neurotransmission of GABA—inducing sleepiness (Mwebe 2021).

Melatonin

Melatonin is only licensed for people over the age of 55 in the UK. Melatonin is a naturally occurring hormone, made by the pineal gland. It helps by helping the body to recognise sleep and waking. As we age, this melatonin naturally reduces and so

Table 4 Side effects of melatonin

Common	Uncommon	Rare or very rare
Arthralgia Increased risk of infection Pain	Anxiety Asthenia Chest pain Dizziness Drowsiness	

Table 5 Side effects of anxiolytics

Benzodiazepines	Buspirone
Rapid onset	Delayed onset
Can induce sedation	Does not have sedating effects
Drug interaction with CNS depressants	Non-addictive
Falls risk	No interaction with CNS depressants
May impair performance	Does not impair performance

consuming pharmacological supplements of the hormone can increase natural capacity to promote sleep (Mwebe 2021). The side effects of melatonin are included in Table 4 (Mwebe 2021; NICE 2024).

Non-Benzodiazepine Anxiolytics

Non-benzodiazepine anxiolytics include buspirone and beta blockers, antidepressants, antipsychotics and anticonvulsants. Buspirone is thought to be less sedating than other anxiolytics, although has a slow onset of action. However, unlike other similar medications, it does not normally lead to dependence issues or have any withdrawal symptoms (Mwebe 2021). Within Table 5, the side effects of benzodiazepines and buspirone are identified (Mwebe 2021).

Antipsychotics

Antipsychotics have typically been split into two different categories, typical and non-typical antipsychotics, which have been broken down in Table 6 (NICE 2025).

Typical Antipsychotics

Typical antipsychotics (or first generation) antipsychotics are antipsychotics that work on the dopamine D2 receptor antagonism. These are drugs that have been available since the 1960s, and are mainly used to treat schizophrenia, organic psychosis and mania (Lyman and McCutcheon 2025). Typical antipsychotics are still a

Table 6 Common antipsychotic drugs

Oral first generation (typical)	Oral second generation (atypical)	Antipsychotic depot injections
Benperidol	Amisulpride	Apriprazole
Chlorpromazine	Aripiprazole	Flupentixol Decanoate
Fluphenazine Decanoate	Asenapine	Fluphenazine Decanoate
Flupentixol	Cariprazine	Haloperidol
Haloperidol	Clozapine	Olanzapine embonate
Levomepromazine	Lurasidone hydrochloride	Paliperidone
Pericyazine	Olanzapine	Pipotiazine Palmitate
Perhenazine	Paliperidone	Risperidone
Pimozide	Quetiapine	Zuclopenthixol decanoate
Prochlorperazine	Risperidone	
Promazine		
Sulpride		
Trifluoperazine		
Zuclopenthixol		

key treatment pathway in mental health services and offer an alternative when second-generation (atypical) medications are not tolerated well.

Typical antipsychotics bind strongly to D2 receptors in the mesolimbic pathway to provide the antipsychotic effects. They also bind to receptors elsewhere in the brain. This includes areas of the brain involved in motor movement, such as the basal ganglia and cerebellum. This means some of the adverse effects including tremors, akinesia (slowing of voluntary movements), spasticity, akathisia (restlessness in legs), and rigidity. These are motor dysfunctions that you may relate to Parkinson's disease. Tardive dyskinesia is another common side effect in typical antipsychotics—where people experience involuntary, disruptive and repetitive body movements.

Typical antipsychotics also may interfere with endocrine function and can induce different cardiovascular effects, sedation and antimuscarinic effects (constipation, dry mouth, nausea, vomiting and dyspepsia). Other side effects that may be commonly seen with these antipsychotics in apathy, amotivation and anhedonia.

Atypical Antipsychotics

The newer atypical antipsychotics include drugs such as clozapine, risperidone, olanzapine, quetiapine, and amisulpride (Blows 2010). Atypical antipsychotics are often referred to as second-generation antipsychotics. These are drugs that have a lower affinity for the D2 receptors, and this in turn reduces the risk of movement disorders (Mwebe 2021). Atypical antipsychotics are better tolerated than first-generation antipsychotics in overdose and they cause fewer extra-pyramidal side effects (Mwebe 2021).

Table 7 Examples of atypical antipsychotic drugs

Atypical antipsychotic drugs	Indication	Oral Dose
Aripiprazole	Mania; short-term management of acute psychosis	10–30 mg
Clozapine	Treatment resistant schizophrenia	Starting dose of 12.5 mg up to 900 mg. Therapeutic dose normally between 200 and 450 mg.
Olanzapine	Schizophrenia; mania; short-term management of acute psychosis; mania	5–20 mg
Quetiapine	Schizophrenia; bipolar disorder; mania	50–800 mg
Risperidone	Schizophrenia; bipolar disorder; mania	1–16 mg

Clozapine

Clozapine is maybe one of the most well-known atypical antipsychotic drugs and is also known for being very effective. It has low side effects and high efficacy (Blows 2010). However, this is a drug treatment only used for those people with schizophrenia who have not responded to other drug treatments (Blows 2010). This is due to one potential side effect—dyscrasia. Dyscrasia is a serious disturbance to the number of blood cells in circulation, which causes a dangerous fall in the leukocyte count (Blows 2011). Service users on clozapine have to be treated by a specialist and be registered on a special monitoring system (Blows 2010).

Some of the more common atypical antipsychotics and their dosage have been included in Table 7 (Mwebe 2021).

Atypical drugs are associated with a range of side effects (Table 7), including glycaemic abnormalities, dyslipidaemias and weight gain. This is thought to be partly due to complex psychodynamic effects of atypical antipsychotics on receptors in the body. Histaminergic transmission on histamine receptors is involved in energy homeostasis and is involved in key roles such as appetite, sleep/wake cycles, learning and sexual behaviours. Histamine also decreases appetite and controls frequency of eating. H1 receptor antagonism by antipsychotics (e.g. haloperidol, chlorpromazine, quetiapine, clozapine and olanzapine) has been found to be the biggest predictor of weight gain and increased energy intake (Mwebe 2021).

Monitoring Requirements

There are several requirements in monitoring of antipsychotics. Weight should be measured at the start of therapy with antipsychotics and then measured weekly for the first 6 weeks. Weight should also be measured at the 12-week mark, and after 1 year. Yearly weight monitoring should continue when people have been established on antipsychotics (NICE 2025).

Fasting blood glucose, Hba1c, and blood lipid concentrations should also be measured at baseline, at 12 weeks, and at 1 year. These should be continued on a yearly basis. Prolactin concentrations are also measured at baseline (NICE 2025).

Before initiating an antipsychotic medication, an ECG may be advised. This may be essential for those service users who have cardiovascular risk factors or family/ personal history of cardiovascular disorders. An ECG is also routinely done on admission to an inpatient unit (NICE 2025).

Neuroleptic Malignancy Syndrome

Neuroleptic Malignant Syndrome (NMS) is a potentially life-threatening reaction to neuroleptic medications such as those to treat psychosis.

Symptoms include:

- Fever.
- Muscle rigidity.
- Altered metal status—confusion, agitation or altered consciousness.
- Alterations to the autonomic nervous system.
- Hyperthermia.
- Autonomic instability.

NMS is most common after starting or increasing the dose of these types of medications, normally within 10 days of this happening.

The management of NMS needs to be immediate and breathing and airways should be protected. It is best to avoid physical restraint as this can worsen the hyperthermia. Medical advice should be sought to support with the withdrawal of neuroleptic drugs (Health Education England n.d.-a).

Mood Stabilisers

The use of mood-stabilising medication is often seen when someone is being treated for bipolar disorder. Bipolar disorder can respond well to medication; however, often more than one medication is used to achieve this effect. This means those with a bipolar disorder often are involved in 'polypharmacy' (Holland 2022).

Five key medications are used as mood-stabilising drugs within the UK, which are the following:

- Lithium.
- Valproate.
- Carbamazepine.
- Lamotrigine.
- Asenapine (Holland 2022).

Current NICE Guidance (NICE 2024) recommends that Lithium is offered as the first-line, long-term pharmacological treatment. If this is unsuccessful or poorly tolerated, an antipsychotic should be recommended (e.g. asenapine, aripiprazole, olanzapine, quetiapine or risperidone).

Lithium

Lithium is a natural mineral, rather than a pharmaceutical drug (Holland 2022).

Lithium is another medication (similarly to Clozapine) that has special monitoring processes due to the risk and side effects associated. Those started on lithium will be assigned a lithium treatment pack to keep monitoring on track and to provide a record of monitoring. This is normally a purple pack and contains a booklet in which all blood tests can be recorded and a lithium alert card, and a lithium information booklet (Holland 2022).

Task

Some organisation will use their own booklets or monitoring documents. Have a look into your own local organisations to see what monitoring documents you use locally.

All service users will have regular blood tests to assess lithium levels, which is how much lithium is in their blood. Lithium has a very narrow window for safe use—0.4–1.0 mmol/L (Holland 2022). Lithium rates can be impacted by metabolic rate, salt intake, weight, and exercise levels. Until a safe level is reached, service users may need to make lifestyle adjustments that could impact fluid balances and salt intake (Holland 2022).

Lithium toxicity may be reached when a person goes higher than 1.5 mmol/L. This may happen at any time in a person taking lithium, and any concerns about lithium toxicity must be acted upon quickly. Lithium toxicity can be fatal (Holland 2022).

Lithium toxicity can present with key symptoms as indicated in Fig. 2 (Holland 2022):

There are a number of contraindications for lithium:

- Addison's disease.
- Cardiac disease—associated with rhythm disorder.
- Cardiac insufficiency.
- Dehydration.
- Family history of Brugada syndrome or personal history of Brugada syndrome.
- Low sodium diets.
- Untreated hypothyroidism.

There are also a number of known side effects of lithium which have been included in Table 8 (NICE 2025).

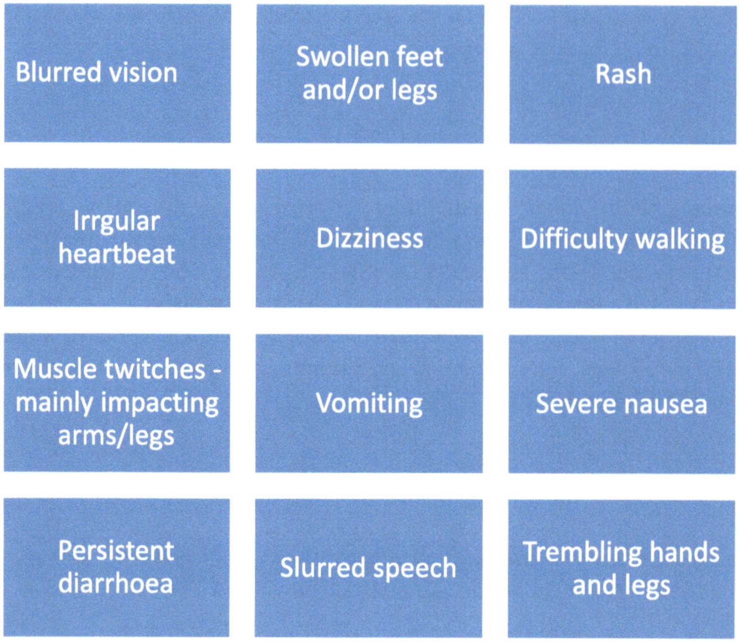

Fig. 2 Lithium toxicity signs and symptoms

Table 8 Side effects of lithium

Common	Rare of very rare
Electrolyte imbalance	Nephrotic syndrome

Asenapine

Asenapine is an antipsychotic medication but is not currently used as an antipsychotic in UK practise; it is purely used for mood stabilisation (Holland 2022).

Asenapine is licensed in the UK for use by sublingual administration. The normal adult dose is 5 mg twice daily and can be increased to 10 mg twice daily if required (Joint Formulary Committee 2026a).

Valproate

Semi sodium valproate is licensed in the UK for the treatment of acute mania, although this is not licensed for use with children. Sodium valproate and valproic acid are not licensed for use in bipolar (Joint Formulary Committee 2026b).

There are a number of contraindications and cautions for the use of bipolar:

- Valproate should not be prescribed with caution to those with systemic lupus erythematosus.
- It should not be prescribed to those with active liver disease; personal or family history of severe, drug-related, hepatic dysfunction; acute porphyria; mitochondrial enzyme polymerase (polg), for example Alpers–Huttenlocher Syndrome.

Women and girls of childbearing potential should not be prescribed valproate. Valproate is a teratogen and can cause significant physical birth defects and developmental disorders in children exposed in utero. Females of childbearing potential taking valproate should be enrolled in a pregnancy prevention plan.

People under the age of 55 (including males) should only be initiated on valproate if two independent specialists have considered and documented that there is no suitable alternative treatment. Evidence has suggested that valproate use in men around the time of conception can affect the neurodevelopment of a child (NICE 2014).

There are a number of adverse effects of valproate:

- Gastric irritation.
- Hyperammonaemia.
- Lethargy and confusion.
- Weight gain.
- Hair loss.
- Peripheral oedema.
- Hyperpigmentation.
- Fulminant hepatic failure—rare.
- Hyperandrogenism in women.
- Thrombocytopenia; leucopoenia; red cell hypoplasia.
- Pancreatitis.
- Small risk of suicidal thoughts and behaviours.
- Severe cutaneous adverse reactions (SCARs) such as Stevens–Johnson syndrome; toxic epidermal necrolysis; drug reaction with eosinophilia and systemic symptoms (NICE 2014).

Key drug interactions of valproate:

- Highly protein-bound drugs may displace valproate from albumin and precipitate toxicity (e.g. aspirin).
- Other less strongly protein-bound drugs can be displaced by valproate and can lead to higher free levels and increased therapeutic effects of toxicity of the concomitant drug (e.g. warfarin).
- Drugs that inhibit cytochrome P450 enzymes (e.g. fluoxetine) can increase valproate levels.
- Valproate can increase the plasma levels of some drugs (e.g. clomipramine).
- Nimodipine—Levels of this drug can be increased when taken with valproate.

- Lamotrigine—Valproate increases the exposure to lamotrigine.
- Carbapenem antibiotics (e.g. imipenem) decrease in blood levels of valproic acid.
- Quetiapine can increase risk of neutropenia and leucopoenia (Joint Formulary Committee 2026c; NICE 2014)

When you are working with someone who is taking valproate, you should be particularly careful to look for signs and symptoms of blood disorders, liver disorder and pancreatitis (Joint Formulary Committee 2026c).

Carbamazepine

UK brand names include: Carbogen SR, Tegretol, Tegretol Retard and Teril Retard.

Carbamazepine is another of the anticonvulsant medications. It comes in liquid and tablet form.

Key drug interactions of carbamazepine:

- MAOI antidepressants—carbamazepine must not be taken with any MAOI antidepressants.
- St John's Wort—It must not be taken with this over-the-counter medication.
- Advice should be sought if a person is taking other medicines for epilepsy, anticoagulants, omeprazole, any psychotic medication, any antidepressant medication, medicine used to treat sickness, antibiotics, water tablets, hormone replacement therapy (HRT), antifungals, corticosteroids, painkillers, asthma medicines, oral contraceptives (efficacy of these can be decreased), levothyroxine, medicines for cancer, medicines for HIV, bupropion, antihistamines and vitamin B supplements (Holland 2022).

Lamotrigine

UK brand names include: Lactimal.

Lamotrigine is another of the anticonvulsant medications. It comes in liquid and dispersible tablet.

Advice should be sought if the medication is taken with:

- Epilepsy medication.
- Olanzapine.
- Risperidone.
- Lithium.
- Aripiprazole.
- Carbamazepine.
- Bupropion.
- Rifampicin.

- Medicines for HIV.
- Oral contraceptives (Holland 2022).

Drugs for Dementia/Delirium

Evidence-based recommendations advise donepezil, galantamine, rivastigmine and memantine for treating Alzheimer's disease.

The two acetylcholinesterase (AChE) inhibitors (donepezil, galantamine and rivastigmine) are recommended for use in managing mild to moderate Alzheimer's disease. Memantine monotherapy is recommended as an option for managing Alzheimer's disease for people with moderate Alzheimer's disease who are intolerant of or have a contraindication for AChE inhibitors or severe Alzheimer's Disease (NICE 2018).

Antipsychotic drugs should only be offered if service users are at risk of harming themselves or others, or experiencing extreme agitation, hallucinations or delusions that are causing distress. The balance and risks should be carefully assessed, including previous history of strokes, transient ischaemic attacks and risk factors for hypertension, diabetes, smoking or atrial fibrillation (NICE 2018).

Adherence and Concordance

Non-adherence should not be seen as a service user issue, but something that needs further exploration. There are two different causes of non-adherence, but they fall into two categories: intentional and unintentional (NICE 2009). Unintentional non-adherence occurs when people cannot follow the adherence plan due to factors outside of their control. This might include things such as problems with using the treatment or forgetting to take the medication. Intentional non-adherence occurs when a service user decides not to follow the treatment recommendations. This might be because of their beliefs or preferences about a treatment plan (NICE 2009).

Depots

Depot antipsychotics are commonly used to improve adherence and clinical outcomes (such as relapse or admission) (Kisely et al. 2015). All depot medications are given as intramuscular injections. These are routinely given in the dorsogluteal area, although the ventrogluteal site is also becoming a popular alternative (Holland 2022).

Some people may have made a personal choice to have an injection rather than take a daily medication, others may be on a depot injection due to concerns about compliance (Holland 2022). For some people, taking a daily medication may remind them of their illness and be an unwelcome reminder of their mental health. They may like the opportunity to have an injection once a month and to forget about it. In some cases, this depot injection can be done in the GP surgery, much like a contraceptive medication. Others may prefer to take a daily pill.

Antipsychotic medication that are available as depot injections are:

- Aripiprazole.
- Flupentixol decanoate.
- Fluphenazine decanoate.
- Haloperidol.
- Olanzapine embonate.
- Paliperidoen.
- Pipotiazine Palmitate.
- Risperidone.
- Zuclopenthizol Decanoate (Joint Formulary Committee 2026d).

A 2015 study completed a systematic review looking at whether the frequency of depot antipsychotic administration (2 vs 4 weekly) makes any difference to compliance and outcome. Results of this showed that there were no differences in psychotic symptoms or quality of life between two and four weekly doses. The only significant difference detected was that two weekly injections were less likely to lead to site pain (Kisely et al. 2015).

CTO's

Some people may be under a Community Treatment Order (CTO), although the recent changes in the MHA (MHA 2025) mean that these will have a stricter criterion and require input of community clinician.

CTO was introduced in 2008 and was intended to cater for service users who are 'revolving door' or have recurrent admissions. A CTO is only an option for those on a Section 3. Once a CTO is in place, a service user can be recalled to hospital for up to 72 hours if you are not meeting the conditions of your CTO. CTOs can involve conditions such as living at a certain place, attending activities or therapies, attending appointments or receiving depot injection.

Non-Pharmacological Interventions

Many of the current NICE guidelines offer both guidance for pharmacological and non-pharmacological treatments. Please see Table 9 for a summary of non-pharmacological options mentioned in NICE guidelines for depression, schizophrenia and anxiety (NICE 2022).

We have discussed a number of non-pharmaceutical treatments for mental health so far within this book, including therapies and social prescribing. In this section, we will expand on our summary of non-pharmacological treatments used in mental health services.

Table 9 Non-pharmacological interventions

Depression (NG222)	Guided self-help including structured cognitive behavioural therapy (CBT), structured behavioural activation (BA), problem-solving or psychoeducation Group cognitive behavioural therapy (CBT) Group behavioural activation Individual CBT Individual behavioural activation Group exercise Group mindfulness and meditation Interpersonal psychotherapy Counselling Short-term psychodynamic psychotherapy Individual problem-solving Behavioural couples therapy
Schizophrenia (CG178)	Cognitive behavioural therapy Family intervention Arts therapy
Generalised anxiety disorders (CG113)	Low intensity psychological interventions Individual non-facilitated self-help Cognitive behavioural therapy Applied relaxation

Electroconvulsive Therapy (ECT)

ECT is given to a service user under intravenous sedation or general anaesthesia, and was first used in 1938 (Kennedy et al. 2009). During ECT, small electrical current pulses between 0.5 and 0.9 are applied to trigger seizures. This is thought to alter the concentration of neurotransmitters like GABA and monoamines such as norepinephrine, serotonin, and dopamine (Odermatt et al. 2025).

UK NICE guidelines suggest that ECT is only recommended to achieve rapid and short-term improvement of severe symptoms after trial of other treatment options has been ineffective. TECT is used for individuals with catatonia and prolonged or severe manic episodes. ECT is only given after a documented assessment of risks and potential benefits to the individual.

ECT may cause short- or long-term memory impairment for past events and current events. As this can also be a symptom of many mental health problems, it can be hard to differentiate the effects of ECT from the condition. Other potential complications can be status epilepticus, laryngospasm and peripheral nerve palsy (NICE 2009).

Cognitive Behavioural Therapy

Cognitive behavioural therapy arose from the work of Beck, in the late 1950s. Beck was known to develop cognitive therapy, something we now know as cognitive behavioural therapy. Cognitive behavioural therapy should be thought of as a science and a therapist must adhere to a strict evidence-based approach (Davies et al. 2025).

Beck (1976) outlined three levels of cognition:

- Core beliefs.
- Dysfunctional assumptions.
- Negative automatic thoughts.

Core beliefs are deeply held beliefs about us, others, and the wider world. They are normally learned early in childhood and are influenced by childhood experiences. The cognitive triad of negative core beliefs captures the relationship between core beliefs and self, the world and the future (Fenn and Byrne 2013).

In CBT, the 'cognitive' model is used as the basic framework to understand a person's current distress. This provides the formulation we discussed earlier in this book. CBT aims to teach service users to be their own therapists by changing the way people think and behave. CBT also involves mutually agreed goal setting which should be 'SMART' in nature (specific, measurable, achievable, realistic and time-limited). CBT is a structured and time-limited treatment (Westbrook et al. 2013; Fenn and Byrne 2013).

CBT has been proven to be effective for mental health conditions. A review of meta-analyses comparing CBT to placebo, wait list and no treatment found CBT to be an effective treatment for adult and adolescent bipolar, generalised anxiety, panic disorder, post-traumatic stress disorder, social phobia, childhood depressive and anxiety disorder (Butler et al. 2006). Furthermore, a randomised controlled trial completed in the UK with service users across 18–75 years found that cognitive behavioural therapy is clinically effective and cost-effective for those using it as an adjunct to care that involves antidepressants and when their depression has not responded to pharmacotherapy (Wiles et al. 2016).

DBT

Dialectical behaviour therapy (DBT) is a comprehensive, evidence-based treatment for personality disorder (Swales and Heard 2024; Chapman 2006). DBT has similarities with other cognitive approaches, but there are aspects of DBT that are specific to DBT including:

- The, very specific, five functions of treatment (enhancing capabilities, generalising capabilities, improving motivation and reducing dysfunctional behaviours, enhancing and maintaining therapist capabilities and motivation, and structuring the environment.
- Biosocial theory and focussing on emotions in treatment.

- Dialectical philosophy.
- Acceptance and mindfulness (Chapman 2006).

The overall goal of DBT is to help clients move towards a 'life worth living'. In Table 10 below, you can see an example of components of DBT (UCL 2025; NHS Highland 2025; Swales and Heard 2024; Chapman 2006).

A randomised control trial methodology was used to compare DBT to treatment as usual (TAU) in individuals with cluster B personality disorders. Both DBT and TAU groups improved on the range of measures employed, but the DBT group showed a slightly greater decrease in CORE-OM risk scores, suicidality, and post-traumatic stress disorder severity. Another study was completed in the use of DBT skills programme for drug and alcohol services. The DBT-informed programme was associated with improvements in emotion regulation, increased recovery from substance misuse and a reduction in psychological distress (Heathcote et al. 2024).

Table 10 Common components of DBT therapy

Mode	Functions	Structure	Targets
Individual therapy	Improve motivation	Weekly 45- to 60-minutes sessions	Reduce life-threatening behaviours Reduce therapy interfering behaviours Reduce quality of life interfering behaviours Improve behavioural skills
Skills training	Enhance capabilities	Weekly	Reduce therapy destroying behaviours Reduce therapy interfering behaviours Improve behavioural skills
Phone consultations	Skills generalisation	As needed	Reduce crisis behaviours Improve skill generalisation to natural environment Improve therapeutic alliance
Consultation team	Improve therapist motivation and capabilities	As needed	Improve therapist motivation Improve therapist capabilities Reduce therapist burnout
Multiple	Structure the environment	As needed	Improve reinforcement of adaptive behaviour Reduce punishment of adaptive behaviour Improve other effective contingencies of behaviour

Recovery Colleges

Recovery colleges provide personalised educational mental health support for people who self-refer. They offer an option for a new form of personalised educational mental health support and offer an opportunity to develop a different relationship between services and local communities. Recovery colleges offer key principles of coproduction and codelivery (Allard et al. 2024).

A study looking at one UK recovery college found that 84/101 students completed the course, and no participants were referred for specialist mental health support whilst students. The findings demonstrated the largest self-reported pre–post dataset for students who attended a recovery college (Allard et al. 2024). The RECOLLECT study is a 5-year study looking at the effectiveness and cost-effectiveness of Recovery Colleges and identifying organisational influences and improvements in mental health outcomes. We are awaiting the results of this much bigger study to see how the work of Recovery Colleges could be developed going forward (Hayes et al. 2022).

Key Learning Points

Medication is an important part of mental health practice and is often the foundation of long-term mental health treatment. However, there is also great value in looking at treatment options away from mental health practice.

It is important that we have knowledge of some of the more common medications we may see in practice. There are often drug interactions, side effects and physical monitoring requirements that may be useful to understand in our own scope of practice.

We will likely all come across service users on some medication which requires increased monitoring. It is important we understand what the red-flag symptoms may be with these medications and know what to do.

It is important that we look at non-adherence in a person-centred and holistic way. Non-adherence is often about barriers, and it is important that we take the time to explore what these might be with our service users.

Non-pharmacological interventions are important components of evidence-based care. There is a range of therapies used within mental health services, and having some knowledge of this may help us support our service users better.

Conclusion

This chapter has explored pharmacological and non-pharmacological treatments available within mental health services, emphasising the importance of selecting interventions that are safe, evidence based and responsive to individual need. Whilst pharmacological treatments provide essential symptom relief and play a critical role in managing acute episodes, relapse prevention and long-term stability, they are most effective when delivered as part of a wider therapeutic plan. The non-pharmacological approaches outlined—ranging from psychological therapies to sensory modulation and social prescribing—reinforce the principle that recovery extends beyond symptom reduction. Instead, recovery involves supporting individuals to rebuild identity, reconnect with meaningful activity and regain control over their lives. Recovery-focused care also acknowledges that progress is not always linear and that individuals may require varying levels of support at different stages of their journey.

Throughout this chapter, a consistent theme has been the significance of collaborative working and shared decision-making. This includes discussing potential side effects openly, weighing risks and benefits, acknowledging previous treatment experiences and respecting each person's values and goals. Engaging service users in these conversations strengthens therapeutic relationships and improves adherence to both pharmacological and non-pharmacological interventions. It also promotes empowerment and autonomy, allowing individuals to feel heard, respected and actively involved in shaping their care. Family members, carers and wider support networks may also play an important role in supporting treatment and recovery where appropriate and with consent.

The integration of biological, psychological and social perspectives remains central to modern mental health care. Practitioners must therefore remain flexible, reflective and informed by current evidence, adapting care plans as an individual's needs and preferences evolve. No single intervention can meet all needs, and safe practice requires ongoing monitoring, interdisciplinary collaboration and a commitment to person-centred care. Cultural sensitivity and awareness of health inequalities are also essential in ensuring equitable and accessible treatment for diverse populations.

Ultimately, the combination of medication knowledge, understanding of non-pharmacological strategies and skilled communication equips practitioners to provide holistic, effective and compassionate support. By drawing on multiple approaches, clinicians can better support individuals to achieve stability, autonomy, and long-term wellbeing whilst promoting hope, resilience and meaningful recovery.

References

Allard J, Pollard A, Laugharne R, Coates J, Wildfire-Roberts J, Millward, M, Shankar R (2024). Evaluating the impact of a UK recovery college on mental well-being: pre- and post-intervention study. BJPsych open 10(3):e87. https://doi.org/10.1192/bjo.2023.646. Accessed 3 Jan 2026

Beck AT (1976) Cognitive therapy and the emotional disorders. International Universities Press

Blows WT (2022) The biological basis of mental health. 4th edn. London: Routledge

Blows WT (2010) The biological basis of mental health nursing. 2nd edn. London: Routledge

Butler AC, Chapman JE, Forman EM, Beck AT (2006) The empirical status of cognitive-behavioral therapy: a review of meta-analyses. Clin Psychol Rev 26(1):17–31. https://doi.org/10.1016/j.cpr.2005.07.003. Accessed 10 Mar 2026

Chapman AL (2006) Dialectical behavior therapy: current indications and unique elements. Psychiatry (Edgmont (Pa.&space;: Township)), 3(9):62–68

Davies J, Salkovskis P, Laidlaw K (2025) An Overview of the Model. In: Cambridge Guide to Cognitive Behavioural Therapy (CBT). Cambridge Guides to the Psychological Therapies. Cambridge University Press; 1–36

Fenn K, Byrne M (2013) 'The key principles of cognitive behavioural therapy', InnovAiT 6(9):579–585. Available at: https://doi.org/10.1177/1755738012471029. Accessed 3 Jan 2026

Hayes D, Henderson C, Bakolis I, Lawrence V, Elliott RA, Ronaldson A, Richards G, Repper J, Bates P, Brewin J, Meddings S, Winship G, Bishop S, Emsley R, Elton D, McNaughton R, Whitley R, Smelson D, Stepanian K, McPhilbin M, Dunnett D, Hunter-Brown H, Yeo C, Jebara T, Slade M. (2022) Recovery Colleges Characterisation and Testing in England (RECOLLECT): rationale and protocol. BMC Psychiatry. Sep 24;22(1):627. https://doi.org/10.1186/s12888-022-04253-y. PMID: 36153488; PMCID: PMC9509550. Accessed 3 Jan 2026

Heathcote D, MacDonald-Winship L, Brown A, Lord S, Marsh D, Dalrymple, L, Huke K (2024) Managing emotions: A service evaluation of a dialectical behaviour therapy (DBT) informed skills group within community drug and alcohol services. Clin Psychol Forum 382:47–54. Available at: https://doi.org/10.53841/bpscpf.2024.1.382.47. Accessed 3 Jan 2026

Health Education England (n.d.-a) NMS. Available at: https://www.hee.nhs.uk/sites/default/files/documents/NMS.pdf. Accessed 7 May 2026

Health Education England (n.d.-b) Serotonin syndrome: clinical guidance. Available at: https://www.hee.nhs.uk/sites/default/files/documents/Serotonin_Syndrome.pdf. Accessed 30 Mar 2026

Holland EJ (2022) The nurse's guide to mental health medicines, 2nd edn. SAGE Publications, London

Johnson CF, Maxwell M, Williams, B, Dougall N, MacGillivray S (2022) Dose-response effects of selective serotonin reuptake inhibitor monotherapy for the treatment of depression: systematic review of reviews and meta-narrative synthesis. BMJ Medicine 1(1):e000017. https://doi.org/10.1136/bmjmed-2021-000017. Accessed 3 Jan 2026

Joint Formulary Committee (2026a) Lithium carbonate. British National Formulary (BNF). NICE. Available at: https://bnf.nice.org.uk/drugs/lithium-carbonate/. Accessed 30 Mar 2026

Joint Formulary Committee (2026b) Sodium valproate. British National Formulary (BNF). NICE. Available at: https://bnf.nice.org.uk/drugs/sodium-valproate/. Accessed 2 May 2026

Joint Formulary Committee (2026c) Quetiapine. British National Formulary (BNF). NICE. Available at: https://bnf.nice.org.uk/drugs/quetiapine/. Accessed 8 February 2026

Joint Formulary Committee (2026d) Antidepressant drugs. British National Formulary (BNF). NICE. Available at: https://bnf.nice.org.uk/treatment-summaries/antidepressant-drugs/. Accessed 30 Mar 2026

Kennedy SH, Milev R, Giacobbe P, Ramasubbu R, Lam RW, Parikh SV, Patten SB,Ravindran AV (2009) Canadian network for mood and anxiety treatments (CANMAT) clinical guidelines for the management of major depressive disorder in adults. IV. Neurostimulation therapies. J Affect Disord 117:S44–53

Kim J, De Jesus O (2023) Medication routes of administration. In: StatPearls [Internet]. Treasure Island (FL): StatPearls Publishing. Available at: https://www.ncbi.nlm.nih.gov/books/NBK568677/. Accessed 8 July 2026

Kisely S, Sawyer E, Robinson G, Siskind D (2015) A systematic review and meta-analysis of the effect of depot antipsychotic frequency on compliance and outcome, Schizophr Res 166(1–3):178–186. https://doi.org/10.1016/j.schres.2015.05.006. Accessed 3 Jan 2026.

Lyman M, McCutcheon R A (2025) Antipsychotic drugs at 75: the past, present, and future of psychosis management. Br Med Bull 156(1): ldaf016. Available at: https://doi.org/10.1093/bmb/ldaf016. Accessed 24 July 2026.

Mental Health Act (2025) (c. 33), UK. Available at: https://www.legislation.gov.uk/ukpga/2025/33 Accessed: 18 July 2026

Mwebe H (2021) Psychopharmacology: a mental health professional's guide to commonly used medications, 2nd edn. Critical Publishing, St Albans

National Institute for Health and Care Excellence (NICE) (2018) Dementia. Available at: https://bnf.nice.org.uk/treatment-summaries/dementia/. Accessed 30 Mar 2026

National Institute for Health and Care Excellence (NICE) (2009) CG76 introduction. Available at: https://www.nice.org.uk/guidance/cg76/chapter/Introduction. Accessed 30 Mar 2026

National Institute for Health and Care Excellence (NICE) (2014) Bipolar disorder: assessment and management (CG185). Available at: https://www.nice.org.uk/guidance/cg185/resources/bipolar-disorder-assessment-and-management-pdf-35109814379461. Accessed 30 Mar 2026

National Institute for Health and Care Excellence (NICE) (2022) Depression in adults: treatment and management (NG222). Available at: https://www.nice.org.uk/guidance/ng222/resources/depression-in-adults-treatment-and-management-pdf-66143832307909. Accessed 30 Mar 2026

National Institute for Health and Care Excellence (NICE) (2024) Prolonged-release melatonin | Prescribing information | Insomnia. Clinical Knowledge Summaries. Available at: https://cks.nice.org.uk/topics/insomnia/prescribing-information/prolonged-release-melatonin/. Accessed 10 May 2026

National Institute for Health and Care Excellence (NICE) (2025) Depression: Tricyclic antidepressants – prescribing information. Clinical Knowledge Summaries. Available at: https://cks.nice.org.uk/topics/depression/prescribing-information/tricyclic-antidepressants/. Accessed 3 Jan 2026

NHS Highland (2025) Dialectical Behaviour Therapy (DBT) factsheet. Personality Disorder Integrated Care Pathway. Available at: https://www.rightdecisions.scot.nhs.uk/media/y3zfn5gf/113-dialectical-behaviour-therapy-dbt-factsheet.pdf. Accessed 24 July 2026

Odermatt J, Sarlon J, Schaefer N, Ulrich S, Ridder M, Schneider E, Lang UE, Liwinski T, Brühl AB (2025) Electroconvulsive therapy reduces suicidality and all-cause mortality in refractory depression: A systematic review and meta-analysis of neurostimulation studies. Neurosci Appl 2;4:105520. Available at: https://doi.org/10.1016/j.nsa.2025.105520. PMID: 41323432; PMCID: PMC12664644. Accessed 3 Jan 2026.

Swales M, Heard H (2024) The state of the science: dialectical behavior therapy. Clin Psychol Rev 110:102449. Available at: https://www.sciencedirect.com/science/article/pii/S0005789424000303. Accessed 30 Mar 2026

Thompson D, DiMartini A (1999) Nonenteral routes of administration for psychiatric medications: a literature review. Psychosomatics 40(3):185–192. Available at: https://doi.org/10.1016/S0033-3182(99)71234-X. Accessed 3 Jan 2026

University College London (UCL) (2025) Specific interventions: Adult. UCL Faculty of Brain Sciences. Available at: https://www.ucl.ac.uk/brain-sciences/sites/brain_sciences/files/2025-10/Specific%20interventions-adult.pdf. Accessed 24 July 2026

Westbrook D, Kennerley H, Kirk J (2013) The key principles of cognitive behavioural therapy. Cogn Behav Therap 6(1):1–8. Available at: https://journals.sagepub.com/doi/10.1177/1755738012471029. Accessed 30 Mar 2026

Wiles N, Thomas L, Abel A, Ridgway N, Turner N, Campbell J, Garland A, Hollinghurst S, Jerrom B, Kessler D, Kuyken W, Morrison J, Turner K, Williams C, Lewis G (2016) Long-term effectiveness and cost-effectiveness of cognitive behavioural therapy as an adjunct to pharmacotherapy for treatment-resistant depression in primary care: follow-up of the CoBalT randomised controlled trial. Lancet Psychiatry 3(2):137–144. Available at: https://www.thelancet.com/journals/lanpsy/article/PIIS2215-0366(15)00495-2/fulltext. Accessed 30 Mar 2026

Interprofessional Work

Why Interprofessionalism Matters?

Case Study

Maria is a 38-year-old woman who has a long-standing bipolar disorder and type 2 diabetes. She lives alone and works part-time but recently has experienced a deterioration following the death of her brother. Maria was brought to the GP after neighbours reported she was tearful and confused outside her apartment block. A neighbour who she works with also states that she has not been in work for the last 4 days. During assessment, Maria states she is not sleeping, she feels 'bottom of the bottom', and she is having difficulty remembering to take her medication. Maria states she is also getting alcohol off another neighbour to help her cope.

Looking through her notes, Maria's blood glucose has been unstable over the last 3 months. She has also not attended the last two appointments with the practice nurse. Maria tells you today she is struggling to mobilise as she feels her feet are 'numb' and she doesn't really know why. You see on her notes that she has seen her mental health nurse 2 weeks ago, who states she feels her mood is dropping.

1. What physical health priorities should be addressed during the initial assessment of Maria?
2. How can adult nurses or other professionals work collaboratively with mental health professionals to support Maria's medication adherence?
3. What role can adult nurses play in addressing the risks associated with Maria's increased alcohol use?
4. How might interprofessional teamwork improve Maria's long-term self-management of her diabetes and overall wellbeing?

R. Bage, *Mental Health Skills for Adult Nurses & Non-Specialist Healthcare Workers*, https://doi.org/10.1007/978-3-032-32835-9_10

The literature suggests that the term 'interprofessional' is not a clearly defined concept (Day 2013). Below is a summary of some definitions of interprofessional collaboration and interprofessional practice.

Rawson (1994: 39) identified a number of groupings of terms based on three sets of concepts:

Problematic association—This looks at terms such as inter/multi/trans.
Grouping—Professional/occupational/disciplinary/sectoral/agency.
Focus of operations—Work/teamwork/collaboration/co-operation/integrations.

Green and Johnson (2015) describe that interprofessional collaboration when more than one professional groups work together to achieve a common goal or goals and can be used as an approach to solve a variety of problems.

The World Health Organization defines interprofessional collaboration as multiple health workers from differing professional backgrounds working with service users, families and carers and the wider community to deliver a good quality of care (WHO 2010).

In 2010, the World Health Organization launched a framework for action in IPE and collaborative practice (CP). This identified the importance of pre-registration health care professionals being 'collaborative practice ready'.

Interprofessional practice has been endorsed as a strategy to help develop a high-quality of health service (Cui et al. 2022). Some of the drivers of interprofessional working have included:

The voice of the service user.
Policies.
Poor Collaborative Practice.
Professional developments.
Technological developments (Day 2013).

Service users with mental health challenges are often complex. They may have concurrent mental health, physical health and social, financial or family challenges. Interprofessional practice is also important to ensure people with mental health problems are not detained unnecessarily (Brodwin 2023).

In Maria's case, there is a clear benefit of working interprofessionally. We can see there may be a clear correlation between her mental health deterioration and her physical health. Equally, there is unlikely to be the skillset in one professional to help Maria alone, and the joint expertise from a range of professionals may be needed to ensure that Maria is stabilised.

Who's Who in MH Care?

Psychiatrists

Psychiatry is a branch of medicine dealing with people from a huge range of mental health conditions. Psychiatrists are medically trained doctors who specialise in psychiatry (Royal College of Psychiatrists 2023a). All psychiatrists complete at least 12 months in General Adult psychiatry before going on to train in either one or two specialities:

- Child and Adolescent.
- General Adult.
- Psychotherapy.
- Forensic.
- Old Age.
- Intellectual Disabilities (RCPsych 2023a).

Psychiatry involves the brain, mind, human behaviours and social relationships (Fiorillo and Maj 2018). Psychiatry has traditionally been quite separate from other branches of medicine, which has been influenced by both physical (typically treated in different hospitals/asylums) and conceptual. Traditionally, it was thought you were only suffered with a mental health disorder, and you could not possibly have a physical health problem as well (Fiorillo and Maj 2018).

In many countries, there is a shortage of psychiatrists, and some people are worried about the long-term viability of psychiatrists (Katschnig 2010). The most recent report from the RCPsych suggests there is currently a shortfall of 690 consultant psychiatrists across England, which equates to around 15% of the current consultant psychiatrist workforce (RCPsych 2023b).

Mental Health Nurses

Mental health nurses come from all backgrounds and experiences. My own experience as a lecturer has seen how lucky mental health is to have so many people choose to join the profession because of their own, friends' or families' experiences of poor mental health. We also attract those who are school or college leavers, who have been inspired by family or own experiences, mainstream or social media or courses such as psychology at school/college.

The mental health nurse's handbook was published in 2022 and was designed to give a practical guide to support preceptorship and supervision conversation. It identifies nine key personal qualities of a mental health nurse:

- Be able to listen in a non-judgemental way.
- Self-awareness.
- Be skilled in being alongside those who were distressed, angry, fearful, and vulnerable.

- High level of knowledge about issues, treatments and resources.
- Adopt a flexible communication style.
- Respectful.
- Available.
- Honest.
- Kind (NHS England 2023).

It also goes on to discuss the nursing interventions which are seen to be the most effective and helpful for those who use mental health service users:

- 1:1 time to support and explain clinical, social, practical options for treatment.
- Knowing and advising when to use medication.
- Intervening and identifying when a person needs something and checking they have what they need.
- Knowledge of practical help available—e.g. personal, social relational, physical.
- Signposting to interventions such as distraction, talking therapy and behavioural support.
- Service-user advocacy.
- Collaborative assessments, goal setting and planning.
- Influencing developments that positively impact experience.
- Ensuring physical health needs are met (NHS England 2023).

An article written in 2022 identified that there is often a limited understanding of the roles, identities and capabilities of mental health nurses (Hurley et al. 2022). Historically, there has been the idea that mental health nursing roles are primarily custodial, basic and under the influence of medicine—due to its history of asylum-based care (Wand et al. 2022). However, the role of the mental health nurse is maybe so diverse that it is hard to reduce to a level understandable to read due to the diversity of roles available (Hurley et al. 2022). We know that mental health nurses routinely work in places such as community, prisons, secure centres, A + E departments and wards, inpatient units, secure units, drug and alcohol services and school and education settings. Mental health nurses are everywhere.

Psychologists

Psychology is the study of how people think, how people act, how people react and how people interact. It looks at aspects of behaviour and how thoughts, feeling and motivation impact behaviour (NHS n.d.).

There are several protected titles for practitioner psychologists in the UK, although the job title ‘psychologist’ is not, by itself, protected by the law. Protected titles, regulated by the Health and Care Professions Council (HCPC) for psychologists are as follows:

- Practitioner psychologist.
- Clinical psychologist.

- Counselling psychologist.
- Educational psychologist.
- Sport and exercise psychologist.
- Registered psychologist.
- Forensic psychologist.
- Health psychologist.
- Occupational psychologist (HCPC 2023).

Clinical psychologists usually use direct observation, interviews and techniques such as psychometric testing. Clinical psychologists also have responsibilities within supervision, advice to other professionals, research and service developments. Training is a 3-year taught doctorate programme within the UK, which involves teaching, supervision and a salaried training post (Sims and Cooper 2025; BMJ 2023).

Educational psychologists are employed normally by local authority children's departments but may also work within charities or child and adolescent mental health services (CAMHS). They work in a variety of different ways including observations, interviews and assessments. To get onto an approved doctorate programme, you must have an approved master's degree in educational psychology and at least 1 year's experience working with young people (Sims and Cooper 2025; BMJ 2023).

You may also see the role of assistant psychologists within the NHS or other health services. Assistant psychologists work as part of a multidisciplinary team and could be involved in:

- Carrying out assessments.
- Carrying out observations.
- Contributing to multidisciplinary discussions around diagnosis, treatment, risk assessment and care plans.
- Exploring a service user's background by reading notes.
- Carrying out treatment or intervention programmes.
- Working with carers and families.
- Researching and gathering information.

Assistant psychologists will always be supervised by a registered psychology practitioner who will maintain the overall clinical responsibility for the service users that assistant psychologists work with. Assistant psychologists tend to be employed at an agenda for change band 4 or 5 level (NHS n.d.).

There are many other professionals who you may also see working in mental health services. These include some of the roles below:

Art Therapy

Art therapy is a form of psychotherapy that uses all different types of art media as a form of expression and communication. They may use art as a tool to address emotional issues which may be challenging, confusing, or distressing (NHS Health Careers 2025a).

Drama Therapy

Drama therapy uses tools such as role play, voice work, movement and storytelling to help service users to explore and solve personal and social problems (NHS n.d.).

Music Therapy

These are specialists that use the power of music to help people deal and cope with feelings and emotions that they may struggle to put into words. They can help service users reach therapeutic goals through the development of music and relationships (NHS n.d.).

Occupational Therapy

An occupational therapist working within mental health services will help somebody to adapt to everyday activities such as work or volunteering (NHS n.d.).

Social Work

Social workers will work with people across a range of settings. It could be about ongoing assessment of a service user's needs and arranging ongoing support (NHS 2025).

There is an increasing number of mental health services who are employing 'mental health practitioners' rather than requesting a specific profession. This means there may be social workers, occupational therapists and nurses doing similar roles in mental health places, with a special interest in their own field. For example, in a mental health crisis team, there may be a range of social workers, nurses and occupational therapists employed doing a similar or identical role.

Psychological Wellbeing Practitioners

Psychological wellbeing practitioners (PWPs) are trained to assess and support those with common mental health problems and to manage their recovery. Qualified PWPs provide high volume, low intensity CBT-based interventions as Step 2, for people with mild to moderate depression and anxiety disorders (Health Careers 2025b). They work within NHS Talking Therapies (discussed in chapter 'Healthcare Environments'), which provides evidence-based therapies for people with common mental health problems such as anxiety and depression (Health Careers 2025c).

Training for PWP roles requires on-the-job training and theoretical work—normally around 45 days of academic work over 1 year alongside supervised practice. All training courses for a PWP course must be accredited by the British Psychological Society (BPS) (BMJ 2023).

High-Intensity Workers

The high-intensity therapists offer other therapies such as:

- CBT.
- Counselling.
- Couple Therapy for Depression.
- Brief Dynamic Interpersonal Therapy.
- Interpersonal Psychotherapy (NHS England 2025).

Mechanisms that Work

Reflective Questions
What do you think work is within interprofessional practices?
Have you seen anything that has been particularly effective or ineffective?

If interprofessional is to work, and health and social professionals are to work successfully together, there are three mechanisms which are important to be in action (WHO 2010):

Institutional Support

This shapes the way that people will work together and the difference between constructive collaboration and fragmentation. This requires good governance models, structured protocols and shared operating procedures (SOP's). Equally, it is important that space and time are required for the collaboration to develop and to provide high-quality care.

Working Culture

This is when good interprofessional cultures are developed by establishing structured information systems and processes, good communication and regular dialogue between health and social care procedures.

Environment

This is when space, facilities and the physical environments have been built in a way which supports interprofessional working.

Summary of the Case Study

1. What physical health priorities should be addressed during the initial assessment of Maria?
   The initial assessment should focus on identifying any immediate or life threatening risks to Maria's physical health whilst recognising the impact her mental health may be having on her physical health. You may want to start by doing physical observations, blood work if clinical concerns exist, alcohol use assessment and check basic things such as hydration levels.
2. How can adult nurses or other professionals work collaboratively with mental health professionals to support Maria's medication adherence?
   You may be able to identify some of the barriers to adherence - this could be things such as low mood, memory difficulties or poor motivation.
   Work alongside the GP, mental health nurse and pharmacist to simplify medication regimens where appropriate.
   You may be able to advocate for the use of medication reminders such as dosette boxes, alarms or smartphone apps.
   Professionals may be able to monitor and assess for side effects that may discourage adherence and report concerns promptly.
   Reinforce education about the importance of taking both diabetes and bipolar medications consistently.
   Share information with the appropriate team and service.
3. What role can adult nurses play in addressing the risks associated with Maria's increased alcohol use?
   You may be able to use an alcohol assessment tool within your work enviornment - there is likely to be approved tools within your work policies.
   Explore the reasons for Maria's alcohol use in a non-judgemental manner, recognising that she is using alcohol to cope with grief and worsening mental health.
   Support Maria in using techniques such as motivational interviewing (open ended questions, reflective listening, affirmations, summaries) to encourage different coping strategies.
   Monitor for signs of alcohol withdrawal or physical complications.
   Refer for mental health support or alcohol support services.
4. How might interprofessional teamwork improve Maria's long-term self-management of her diabetes and overall wellbeing?
   Interprofessional working enables Maria's complex physical, psychological and social needs to be addressed simultaneously in a holistic and person-centred way.

Handover

There are several tools that have been shown to be useful in the mental health sphere, that are already used in adult nursing and healthcare practices. Handover processes can often be inconsistent and lacking clear structure, which can compromise clinical safety (Vallabhaneni et al. 2022).

The SBAR tool is one of these tools. This was originally a tool developed by the US Military to allow concise and accurate information to be communicated across a team and reduced likelihood for error (Müller et al. 2018). Standing for Situation–Background–Assessment–Recommendation (SBAR), this tool can be useful for a structured handover (Müller et al. 2018).

Situation—This is when you identify who you are, and where you are calling from. You also need to identify the service user by name and the reason for the referral or phone call. You will need to describe what your concerns are.

Background—This is when you are going to give the background of the admission/attendance and explain any significant medical history. You will also want to give any important detail such as admission date, current medication, allergies and any diagnostic results.

Assessment—This is when you want to give any of the assessment details across including vital signs, clinical impressions and any concerns.

Recommendations—This is where you are going to explain what support you need, and you need to be specific about the period that you need this. You also want to give any suggestions and clarify your expectations from the phone call (Institute for Innovation and Improvement 2010, NHS England 2017).

Referrals Using SBAR

You have two service users within the A + E department who need referring to the Mental Health Liaison Service. Practice with a colleague making these referrals using the SBAR approach.

Kili—Kili is a 23-year-old university student, who was brought to A + E by a friend following disclosure of suicidal thoughts to her friends and making some superficial cuts to her forearms. She reports feeling completely overwhelmed by her current dissertation writing and a deadline coming up next week. In Triage, Kili appears withdrawn, tearful and agitated when someone passes the room. Kili's HR is high, but all other basic observations are normal. Kili has had her arm wounds cleaned and dressed within triage. Kili denies any current intent but is displaying some ambivalence about life. Friends report that she has been worsening over the last 2 weeks after a poor grade at university and they are worried about her. No previous mental health concerns and no known substance misuse. Awaiting a mental health review.

Laurence—Laurence is an 87-year-old male who has been brought to A + E by ambulance. Laurence told a neighbour he 'couldn't go on' and has taken an overdose of his prescribed medication. There is a bit of unclarity in how much medication he has taken as he has a dossette box at home. He reports several weeks of low mood and poor sleep, and he reports having a very low appetite. Laurence lost his wife 4 months ago, and Laurence was her carer. In A + E, he is noted to be very quiet and subdued, and he is actively avoiding any eye contact. He reports hopelessness with the situation and that he 'doesn't want to carry on'. Physical observations are within normal limits, and he has taken no alcohol or illegal drugs. Laurence lives alone and remains physically well. He requires a mental health assessment.

In a study looking to improve mental health service handovers within the integrated liaison assessment team, SBAR was introduced alongside key task allocation and shift handover lead. A regular multidisciplinary team training session was also introduced. Evidence from this study showed 'good' handovers improved and 'poor' rated handovers reduced. Mean handover time also reduced from 47 minutes to 31.25 minutes (Vallabhaneni et al. 2022).

Interestingly, a systematic review looked at the impact of nursing handovers on clinical practice across many settings of health care. The evidence suggested that negative emotions such as stress, anxiety, dissatisfaction and tension are often linked to handovers. Evidence suggested this was often linked to lack of standardised training and consistent practices, often in newly graduated or less experienced nurses. It was found that open communication and supportive environments can help to support team cohesion and reduce stress (Tomás et al. 2025).

Liaison Services: Models and Evidence

Acute Liaison Services

Acute liaison services are designed to provide services to those who are currently in acute settings, inpatient or outpatient, who have, or at risk of a mental disorder. This also includes those in services such as Accident and Emergency Services or Walk in Services (Joint Commissioning Panel for Mental Health 2012).

A 2019 study was completed across 73 liaison psychiatry and acute hospital staff from 11 different acute hospitals in England. There were several key themes found within this work. These included:

- Lack of continuity across secondary-primary interface.
- Lack of mental health services in primary care to support discharge.
- A lack of shared information services.
- A long period of time spent recording information opposed to face-to-face service user contact.
- Lack of shared vision of care (Jasmin et al. 2019).

PLAN is the Psychiatric Liaison Accreditation Network (PLAN), and they facilitate improvement and development in liaison psychiatry services through a peer-review model and enabling communication and sharing of best practice between services. PLAN is open to all liaison mental health services in the United Kingdom.

Quality Standards for Psychiatric Liaison Services—8th Edition (Royal of College of Psychiatrists 2026)

Five Sustainability Principles

Prioritise Prevention

This principle looks at preventing poor mental health and how this can reduce mental health need and reduce the burden on mental health services.

Empower Individuals and Communities

This involves improving the awareness of mental health problems and the importance of promoting opportunities for supporting self-management and independent living. This also looks at ensuring service users and carers are at the centre of the decision-making.

Improve Value

This involves delivering interventions that provide the maximum benefit and at the lowest cost possible and making sure that service users are getting the right intervention at the right time.

Consider Carbon

This requires working with providers to reduce the carbon impacts of interventions and models of care. This also looks at reducing overmedication, adopting a recovery approach, and ensuring nurturing environments are available.

Staff Sustainability

This looks at supporting employees to maintain health and wellbeing. Contributions to the service should be recognised and effective team working facilitated (Royal College of Psychiatrists 2026).

Referrals

One further technique to support referrals to the liaison services is my remember the 'CHIP' acronym for your referrals. C - Current Presentation. This is about making sure you fully explain the current presentation of the person you maybe referring to the Mental Health Liaison team. H - Historic Details. This is ensuring that you are explaining the history of the person - it could be physical health, previous mental health, previous self-harm, or family history of suicide. I - Intention. This is about thinking what your intention is for the referral, or thinking 'what do I want from this?'. It might be behavioural support, psychopharmacology advice, or referral support. It is important to understand what you want and need from a referral. P = Physical Health and Discharge Plan - liaison services will absolutely see service users who are physically unwell, but it is important for liaison services to understand what the current and future plan is. This helps to triage referrals, and to make sure that no service user is waiting on discharge because the liaison services have not yet been able to see them.

Overcoming Friction: Boundaries, Role Clarity, Risk Ownership

Reflective Questions
What do you feel are the frictions in IPE within your workplace?
What friction do you think there is in working with mental health services?

Interprofessional practice should begin in education. Indeed, many of the professional and statutory regulatory bodies for each health and social care profession emphasise the need for students to learn with students from alternative courses (e.g. GMC 2024; HCPC 2025; NMC 2018). A study looking into IPE across Norway and the United Kingdom found four key themes: system approach; curriculum and learning outcomes; person-centred care and professional identity (Lindqvist et al. 2025).

Whole Systems Approach

Results suggested that education leaders agree that a whole systems approach was needed, and this should involve stakeholders including students, clinicians, professional bodies and leaders (Lindqvist et al. 2025).

Curricula

Results suggested that curriculum content linked to IPE required mapping to competencies and evidence-based practice to become truly integrated and not perceived as an 'extra' task. Leadership was important, and it was important that leaders had knowledge of IPE (Lindqvist et al. 2025).

Person-Centred Care

UK participants agreed that focussing on person-centred care would potentially resolve challenges around the integration of IPE into the curriculum and the integration of intercollaborative practice. Practitioners from across the globe felt that bringing students together to solve problems for the service user's benefits was a good pedagogical approach for IPE (Lindqvist et al. 2025).

Professional Identity

Senior leaders across universities considered the importance of professional identity during the development and delivery of IPE. It was also identified that there is an importance in keeping the learning environment safe to ensure students were able to develop their own professional identity (Lindqvist et al. 2025).

Managing Risk

A 2003 study looked at developing, delivering and evaluating interprofessional clinical risk training in mental health services. In this, three different services, two mental health services and one local social services department, were involved in the training. There were four main key objectives re the training:

1. Introduce risk management as a systematic, dynamic process.
2. Outline the link between people with mental disorder and risk.
3. Identify key risk factors.
4. Provide knowledge or risk assessment tools and practice in their use.

A 2-day training format was agreed with four half-day sessions looking at clinical risk management, self-harm and suicide, risk to others and self-neglect.

The satisfaction from this training was 'good' or '3' on the Likert scale. However, common themes emerged across the comments regarding liability for decisions, lack of effective multidisciplinary working, personality disorders, substance misuse, personal safety, limitations of established frameworks, risk management vs. prediction and confidentiality. All participants felt the training had improved their practices in assessment and managing risks (Doyle et al. 2003).

Key Learning Points

Interprofessional practice is an essential part of mental health practice. No single profession can address the overlapping physical, mental health and social needs of service users.

Understanding other professionals' roles can strengthen quality and referrals. There is work we can all do in making sure we have increased knowledge of the role and skillset of other professionals within our multidisciplinary team. There is also reduced friction within teams if we all understand other's roles.

Liaison mental health services can provide a key interface between mental health and physical health services.

There is a significant benefit for service users if the services they are within are well-coordinated and working interprofessionally.

There is value in using structured communication tools to improve our information-sharing within services. You may be well used to tools such as SBAR, and these can be beneficial to use when referring to services such as mental health.

Conclusion

The case of Maria has illustrated how physical health and mental health can be deeply interlinked and woven together. Her case helps us understand how fragmented care can lead to disjointed responses, duplicated assessments, delayed interventions and unmet needs. When professionals work in isolation from one another, important information can be missed, communication may break down and service users may feel unsupported or unheard within the system. Interprofessional care offers us the opportunity to support service users in a deeply holistic way, using shared tools, integrated approaches and consistent language to support the individual throughout their journey. Through collaborative working, professionals are better able to identify risks, coordinate interventions and ensure that care remains focused on the whole person rather than separate diagnoses or services.

Interprofessional practice also brings significant challenges. Professional identity, boundaries, differing approaches to risk and variations in communication styles can all create friction and feelings of discomfort within teams. Organisational pressures, limited resources, and differences in professional priorities may further complicate collaborative working. To address these challenges, practitioners need to be open, reflective and willing to listen to one another. It is important that we understand both our own role and the roles of others within person-centred care, recognising the expertise and contribution each professional brings to the team. Developing mutual respect, psychological safety and shared goals can strengthen teamwork and improve service user outcomes.

High-quality interprofessional practice rests on the understanding that no single professional can meet every need that a service user, their family or carers may have. Effective teamwork therefore becomes essential in ensuring that care is safe, coordinated and responsive to individual needs. Collaborative working also enables practitioners to learn from one another, challenge assumptions, and develop more creative and comprehensive approaches to care planning. By working together and genuinely valuing each other's knowledge, perspectives and experiences, we can ensure that mental health care remains compassionate, person-centred and recovery focused. Ultimately, strong interprofessional relationships not only improve outcomes for service users but also create more supportive and resilient healthcare environments for staff themselves.

References

BMJ Health Careers (2023) The complete guide to becoming a psychologist. Available at: https://www.bmj.com/healthcareers/article/complete-guide-to-becoming-a-psychologist. Accessed 7 May 2026

Brodwin P (2023) Interprofessional learning and psychiatric expertise in mental health courts. AMA J Bus Ethics 25(5):E353–E360. Available at: https://doi.org/10.1001/amajethics.2023.353. Accessed 8 July 2025

Cui J, Newman CE, Lancaster K, Mao L (2022) Interprofessional dynamics that promote client empowerment in mental health practice: a social work perspective. J Soc Work 22(2):364–383. https://doi.org/10.1177/14680173211009714. Accessed 12 March 2026

Day J (2013) Interprofessional working: an essential guide for health and social care professionals. Andover: Cengage Learning

Doyle M, Earnshaw P, Galloway A (2003) Developing, delivering and evaluating interprofessional clinical risk training in mental health services. Psychiatr Bull 27(2):73–76. https://doi.org/10.1192/pb.27.2.73

Fiorillo A, Maj M (2018) The role of psychiatry in modern medicine. Int Rev Psychiatry 30(2):169–175. https://doi.org/10.1080/09540261.2018.1436675. Accessed 12 Nov 2025

General Medical Council (2024) Good medical practice. London: GMC. Available at: https://www.gmc-uk.org/professional-standards/the-professional-standards/good-medical-practice Accessed 12 May 2025

Green BN, Johnson CD (2015) Interprofessional collaboration in research, education, and clinical practice: working together for a better future. J Chiropr Educ 29(1):1–10. https://doi.org/10.7899/JCE-14-36

Health and Care Professions Council (2023) Understanding the regulation of psychologists. Available at: https://www.hcpc-uk.org/news-and-events/blog/2023/understanding-the-regulation-of-psychologists/. Accessed 7 May 2026

Health and Care Professions Council (HCPC) (2025) Standards of education and training. Available at: https://www.hcpc-uk.org/standards/standards-relevant-to-education-and-training/set/ Accessed 12 May 2025

Hurley J, Lakeman R, Linsley P, Ramsay M, McKenna-Lawson S (2022) Utilizing the mental health nursing workforce: a scoping review of mental health nursing clinical roles and identities. Int J Ment Health Nurs 31(4):796–822. https://doi.org/10.1111/inm.12983

Jasmin K, Walker A, Guthrie E, Trigwell P, Quirk A, Hewison J, Murray CC, House A (2019) Integrated liaison psychiatry services in England: a qualitative study of the views of liaison practitioners and acute hospital staff from four distinctly different kinds of liaison service. BMC Health Serv Res 19(1):486. https://doi.org/10.1186/s12913-019-4356-y. Accessed 9 November 2025

Joint Commissioning Panel for Mental Health (2012) Guidance for commissioners of liaison mental health services to acute hospitals. Available at: https://bmjopenquality.bmj.com/content/suppl/2015/04/07/bmjquality.u206661.w2871.DC1/ds4453.pdf. Accessed 7 May 2026

Katschnig H (2010) Are psychiatrists an endangered species? Observations on internal and external challenges to the profession. World Psychiatry 9(1):21–28. https://doi.org/10.1002/j.2051-5545.2010.tb00257.x. Accessed 12 November 2025

Lindqvist S, Wilsher SH, Vasset F, Almås SH, Willumsen E, Iversen HP, Ødegård A (2025) Integrating interprofessional education in health and social care curricula to equip our future workforce—qualitative findings from senior leaders. Soc Sci Humanit Open 12:101236

Müller M, Jürgens J, Redaèlli M, Klingberg K, Hautz WE, Stock S (2018) Impact of the communication and patient hand-off tool SBAR on patient safety: a systematic review. BMJ Open 8(8):e022202. https://doi.org/10.1136/bmjopen-2018-022202. Accessed 12 January 2026

NHS England (2017) Safer care SBAR situation • background • assessment • recommendation: implementation and training guide. NHS England, London. Available at: https://www.england.nhs.uk/improvement-hub/wp-content/uploads/sites/44/2017/11/SBAR Implementation-and-Training-Guide.pdf. Accessed 7 May 2026

NHS England (2023) The mental health nurse's handbook. Available at: https://www.england.nhs.uk/long-read/the-mental-health-nurses-handbook/. Accessed 7 May 2026

NHS England (2025) NHS Talking Therapies: Workforce. Available at: https://www.england.nhs.uk/mental-health/adults/nhs-talking-therapies/workforce/ Accessed 18 July 2025

NHS Health Careers (2025a) Art therapist/art psychotherapist. Available at: https://www.healthcareers.nhs.uk/explore-roles/allied-health-professionals/roles-allied-health-professions/art-therapistart-psychotherapist Accessed 12 May 2025

NHS Health Careers (2025b) Psychological wellbeing practitioner. Available at: https://www.healthcareers.nhs.uk/explore-roles/psychological-therapies/roles-psychological-therapies/psychological-wellbeing-practitioner Accessed: 10 April 2026

NHS Health Careers (2025c) Social worker. Available at: https://www.healthcareers.nhs.uk/explore-roles/wider-healthcare-team/roles-wider-healthcare-team/clinical-support-staff/social-worker. Accessed: 9 July 2026

NHS Institute for Innovation and Improvement (2010) SBAR: Implementation and training guide. Coventry: NHS Institute for Innovation and Improvement. Available at: https://www.england.nhs.uk/improvement-hub/wp-content/uploads/sites/44/2017/11/SBAR-Implementation-and-Training-Guide.pdf Accessed 9 December 2026

Nursing and Midwifery Council (NMC) (2018) The code: professional standards of practice and behaviour for nurses, midwives and nursing associates. Available at: https://www.nmc.org.uk/standards/code/ Accessed 4 January 2026

Rawson D (1994) Models of interprofessional work: likely effects and conditions for success. In: Leathard A (ed) Going Inter-Professional: Working Together for Health and Welfare. London: Routledge, pp 38–49.

Royal College of Psychiatrists (2023a) What is psychiatry? Available at: https://www.rcpsych.ac.uk/become-a-psychiatrist/choose-psychiatry/what-is-psychiatry Accessed: 8 April 2026

Royal College of Psychiatrists (2023b) Royal College of Psychiatrists calls for urgent publication of NHS workforce plan as psychiatrist numbers stagnate. Available at: https://www.rcpsych.ac.uk/news-and-features/latest-news/detail/2023/05/25/royal-college-of-psychiatrists-calls-for-urgent-publication-of-nhs-workforce-plan-as-psychiatrist-numbers-stagnate. Accessed 7 May 2026

Royal College of Psychiatrists (2026) Quality standards for psychiatric liaison services (8th edn). London: Royal College of Psychiatrists. Available at: https://www.rcpsych.ac.uk/docs/default-source/improving-care/ccqi/quality-networks/psychiatric-liaison-services-plan/plan-8th-ed-standards.pdf. Accessed 11 Feb 2025

Sims C, Cooper J (2025) The complete guide to becoming a psychologist. BMJ Health Careers. Available at: https://www.bmj.com/healthcareers/article/complete-guide-to-becoming-a-psychologist Accessed 1 November 2025

Tomás MAR, Soares MR, Oliveira-Lopes JM, Sousa LMM, Martins VLD (2025) The influence of nursing handover on nurses' mental health: a scoping review. AIMS Public Health 12(1):106–123. https://doi.org/10.3934/publichealth.2025008. Accessed 18 January 2026

Vallabhaneni K, Hazan J, Donaldson L, Johansson F (2022) Improving the handover process in a psychiatry liaison setting. BMJ Open Quality 11:e001627. https://doi.org/10.1136/bmjoq-2021-001627 Accessed 12 February 2026.

Wand T, Glover S, Paul D (2022) What should be the future focus of mental health nursing? Exploring the perspectives of mental health nurses, consumers, and allied health staff'. Int J Ment Health Nurs 31(1):179–188. https://doi.org/10.1111/inm.12947. Accessed 14 July 2026

World Health Organization (WHO) (2010) Framework for action on interprofessional education and collaborative practice. Geneva: World Health Organization. Available at: https://iris.who.int/server/api/core/bitstreams/d743ea4e-8c14-493c-b3a5-1a0022e6ce54/content. Accessed: 19 Dec 2025

Inclusivity

The Nursing and Midwifery Council (2021) states clearly that:

> There is no room for any kind of discrimination in the healthcare sector, and we're committed to working with partners to do everything in our power to tackle inequality and promote diversity and inclusion

Reflective Questions
What does inclusivity mean to you?
How do you demonstrate your inclusive practice in your own workplace?

Mental Health Around the World

Mental health continues to disproportionately impact those in our most vulnerable communities (Moitra et al. 2023). Suicide remains illegal in 25 countries, and an additional 20 countries follow Islamic or Sharia law where those who have attempted suicide may be punished with jail sentences (Mishara and Weisstub 2016).

Economic resources play a crucial role in determining the availability and quality of mental health services around the globe, with higher-income countries generally allocating more resources to mental health care. Limiting funding, shortage of mental health trained professionals and inadequate facilities exacerbate the gap between high and low-income countries (Fiorillo et al. 2025). The differences in how mental health is treated across the world impacts how our communities and service users impact mental health care. However, research also suggests that experiences of racism, migration, religion, and complex trauma might be more relevant than ethnic group classifications. Tackling ethnic inequalities in mental healthcare requires an evaluation of individual, systemic, and structural obstacles to authentic and meaningful coproduction and implementation of existing services (Bansal et al. 2022).

R. Bage, *Mental Health Skills for Adult Nurses & Non-Specialist Healthcare Workers*, https://doi.org/10.1007/978-3-032-32835-9_11

Inclusive, Culturally Safe Practice

Culturally appropriate care, or culturally competent care, is care that is sensitive to a person's cultural identity or heritage (CQC 2025). This might be based on ethnicity, nationality, or sexuality or gender identity. People who are deaf who use sign language have a particular culture, as do those who are lesbian, gay, bisexual or transgender (Care Quality Commission 2025).

The United Nations Minorities Declaration refers to minority groups as groups of people who are culturally, racially, religiously or linguistically distinct in a way to many people living within a country or community (United Nations, Human Rights, Office of the High Commissioner 1992).

Inclusion Health

Inclusion is a term used to describe people who are socially excluded and who often experience multiple interacting risk factors for poor health, such as stigma, discrimination and violence (NHS England 2023).

People in inclusion health groups include:

- People who are experiencing homelessness.
- People with drug and alcohol misuse/dependence.
- Vulnerable migrants and refugees.
- Gypsy, Roma and traveller communities.
- People in contact with the justice system.
- Victims involved in modern slavery.
- Those involved in the sex industry (NHS England 2023).

Mulongo and Wainwright (2024) identify six strategies to support mental health nurses develop cultural competency when supporting ethnic minoritised service users, which can be adapted for other clinicians working this patient group.

1. Increasing awareness and education on the cultural and social factors that may impact on the diagnosis and treatment of ethnic minoritised service users. This includes factors such as systemic racism and cultural stigma.
   Clinicians across the health sector need to grow their awareness of how cultural and social factors impact their assessment, treatment and diagnosis of ethnic minoritised service users in all fields. All staff should be aware of how systemic racism and cultural stigma impact the field of mental health.
2. Providing culturally sensitive care that recognises and values the cultural, social and spiritual backgrounds and experiences of service users from ethnic minority backgrounds.
   Clinicians across the health service need to be informed on cultural, social and spiritual backgrounds and know where to go for support if they feel they need further guidance to support patient groups.

3. Considering using culturally appropriate language and interpreters when necessary.
   All staff should feel confident in asking for further guidance re appropriate language and to use interpreters as needed. It can feel uncomfortable to ask questions around suicide and self-harm through interpreters, but it is crucial that you are able to have deep and rich conversations in a way that can be understood.
4. Becoming familiar with specialist agencies to signpost your service users, when necessary, for example, financial support or legal advisors.
   People with mental illness are more likely to need support from other agencies. Please ensure that you are referring, when consent is given, at the earliest opportunity to support this patient group.
5. Being flexible and offering mental health support online, and via helplines, as these may be more convenient for some service users who may have barriers to accessing face-to-face support.
   It is important to ensure that you communicate to mental health professionals when there might be difficulties in accessing face-to-face support. Mental health services have increasingly been providing care in virtual environments as well as face to face. It is important that when discussing mental health with service users, they are made aware that other options may be available if they struggle to access face-to-face care.
6. Advocating for systematic changes that address the root cause of mental health disparities, such as systematic racism.
   All clinicians, whatever their field, should be advocating for this patient group and the systematic challenges such as racism, healthcare structure and the disparities between physical and mental health care.

Race and Mental Health

Race is a protected characteristic under UK Equality Law (Equality Act 2010). Evidence suggests that black and minority ethnic communities are at comparatively higher risk of mental illness and disproportionately impacted by social detriments associated with mental ill health (Bignall et al. 2019).

David 'Rocky' Bennett was a 38-year-old Black Man who had been detained in the Norvic Clinic, Norwich in 1998. Rocky died after being held face down on the floor for 25 minutes by a team of at least four nurses (The Guardian 2004); he was not released until he went quiet and at this point, it was too late. The Inquiry into his death found that staff treated Mr. Bennett as a 'lesser being … who should be ordered about'.

NHS England commissioned a research review as part of the 'Racial Disparities in Mental Health' project. This review found differences in experiences and outcomes of black and minority ethnic people within the white English community (Bignall et al. 2019). Their findings focussed on the topic areas below:

Prevalence

Black and minority ethnic communities are at comparatively higher risk of mental illness. People from African Caribbean communities are more than three times more likely to be diagnosed and admitted to hospital for schizophrenia than any other group (Bignall et al. 2019). Black women are more likely to experience a common mental illness, such as anxiety disorder or depression (Rethink Mental Illness 2025).

There is a lack of consistency within the studies looking into prevalence data, and more work is needed to give us more reliable figures looking into prevalence and mental health (Bignall et al. 2019).

Access

Evidence suggests that black and minority ethnic communities are less likely to access mental health support within primary care services, and therefore, more likely to present in crisis care services (Bignall et al. 2019).

Assessment

Poor health conditions of people in the black and minority ethnic group mean that doctors are more likely to focus on physical health conditions despite there is clear overlap in some conditions. There is no evidence of direct racial discrimination in assessments, but there is evidence of ethnic bias. For example, there is greater evidence of uncertainty by clinicians in the diagnosis of emotional or wellbeing problems and depression in BME services (Bignall et al. 2019).

Treatment

Black and minority ethnic people are less likely to be referred to talking therapies and more likely to be medicated for ill mental health (Bignall et al. 2019). People from most minority ethnic groups are more likely to be detained under the Mental Health Act than the majority white population.

The most recent figures for 2020/21 show the rates of detention were the following:

Black or Black British: 309.4 per 100,000 people
Mixed Ethnicity: 143.9 per 100,000 people
Other ethnic groups: 197.4 per 100,000 people

Asian or Asian British: 96.2 per 100,000 people
White: 76.2 per 100,000 people (NHS Digital 2021)

Recovery

Culture and Mental Health

In 2022, the Mental Health, Learning Disability and Autism Inpatient Quality Transformation Programme was established to support cultural change and remodel care for NHS-funded mental health, learning disability and autism inpatient settings. As part of this, culture of care standards for mental health inpatient care set out a goal for inpatient providers to realise the culture of care for service users, their families and staff. The 12 overarching core commitments are as follows:

1. Lived experience—Value lived experience at all levels including paid roles.
2. Safety—Ensuring that people on our wards feel safe and cared for.
3. Relationships—High-quality, rights-based care starts with trusting relationships and connection.
4. Staff support—Supporting all staff so they can be present alongside people in distress.
5. Equality—Ensuring we are inclusive and value difference. Having a focus on equity.
6. Avoiding harm—Actively seek to avoid harm and traumatisation, and acknowledge the trauma when it happens.
7. Needs led—Respect people's understanding of their distress.
8. Choice—Ensure that people and their carers are engaged in all aspects of their care.
9. Environment—Our inpatient spaces reflect the value we have for people.
10. Things to do on the ward—Wide range of patient requested activities every day.
11. Therapeutic support—Offer people a range of therapy and support that gives people hope.
12. Transparency—Open and honest conversations with service users and each other (NHS England 2025b).

Transcultural Models of Mental Health

There are a number of transcultural models of mental health care. Transcultural psychiatry is a movement that has been developed to address the role of understanding and incorporating the role of culture in psychiatry and mental health care (Ayaz and Asghar-Ali 2025).

Trauma-Informed Care Model (GBV)

Authored by the Substance Abuse and Mental Health Services Administration (2015), it creates a safe and supportive environment, builds trust and empowers service users to make their own choices about their care (Mulongo and Wainwright 2024).

Human Trafficking Intervention Model (HTIM)

This was developed by the University of Pennsylvania School of Nursing in 2014. This highlights a victim-centred approach and provides a safe and supportive environment (Mulongo and Wainwright 2024). Using a transcultural approach can improve assessment and screening processes, which will hopefully support the experience service users get from mental health services. Using this approach may lead to more effective and high-quality care for immigrant and refugee families experiencing mental health disorders (Wylie et al. 2018).

Spirituality in Care

The definition of spirituality is as follows:

> Spirituality is a distinctive, potentially creative and universal dimension of human experience arising both within the subjective awareness of individuals and within communities, social groups, and traditions. It may be experienced as a relationship with that which is intimately 'inner,' immanent and personal, within the self and others, and/or as relationship with that which is wholly 'other,' transcendent and beyond the self. It is experienced as being of fundamental or ultimate importance and is thus concerned with matters of meaning and purpose in life, truth and values. (Cook 2004)

In many cultures, emotional ailments have been considered problems of religious or spiritual origins. Indeed, we know from history that much of the mental health care in the early eras was provided by religious groups (Kao et al. 2020). However, in the early to mid-nineteenth century, mental health and religion and spirituality were viewed very separately (Kao et al. 2020). There is still evidence of religious groups doing significant work in the field of mental health.

There remains a number of theories on why religion, spirituality and mental health may be interlinked:

Relational Spirituality

Relational spirituality is a term that has been increasingly employed in psychology and literature over recent years. Tomlinson et al. (2016) argue that relational spirituality can be understood in five ways:

- Cognitive appraisals of stress and coping.
- Implicit relational development.
- Couples, family and community contexts.
- Social interconnection.
- A differentiation-based model of spiritual development (Tomlinson et al. 2016).

Morality

Research has suggested that excellent character, and adherence to high standards of moral behaviour can contribute to wellbeing. A research study using medical insurance claims found that people who live their life according to high moral standards have substantially lower odds of depression (Weziak-Bialowolska et al. 2023).

A systematic review of the relationship between suicide risk and religion has found that religious affiliation does not necessarily protect against suicidal ideation, and it does protect against suicide attempts. This may be impacted by the cultural-specific implications of being associated with particular religions, as minority groups may become more socially isolated (Lawrence et al. 2016). Most religions prohibit suicide (Gearing and Lizardi 2009).

Spirituality can promote emotional wellness, greater life satisfaction, self-esteem, higher levels of family functioning and better adjustment to clinical concerns (Rosmarin and Koenig 2020).

A meta-analysis was completed on the long-term positive effect of religion or spirituality on mental health. This meta-analysis included 48 longitudinal papers. Results of this showed that of eight factors, only two were shown to have been significantly related to mental health—public religious activities and importance of religion (Garssen et al. 2021). This is not in correlation with earlier studies, which found a much higher association between religious + spirituality and mental health (e.g. Larson et al. 1992).

Gender & LGBTQI+ Considerations

Reflective Questions
How do you support LGBTQI+ service users in your own service?

LGBTQI+

A study by Stonewall found that over the previous year in the UK:

- Half of people identifying as LGBTIQ+ had experienced depression.
- 60% of people identifying as LGBTIQ+ had experienced anxiety.
- Approximately one in eight people aged 18 – 14 identifying as LGBTIQ+ had attempted to end their life.

- Almost half of trans people had thought about ending their life.
- In the most recent National Confidential Inquiry into Suicide and Safety in Mental Health (2026), 5% of mental health service users who died by suicide (National Confidential Inquiry 2026).

LGBTQI+ people experience discrimination, victimisation and lifestyle factors such as alcohol and drugs which increase the risk of morbidity (Cochran 2001; Gibson 1989).

However, lesbian, gay, bisexual, transgender, intersex, queer people and minority gender identities and sexualities are often stigmatised and experience discrimination in healthcare settings (Silveri et al. 2022). People who identify as LGBTQI+ are less likely to access health services and engage with healthcare workers due to stigma or discrimination (World Health Organization 2021). This leads to poorer mental health outcomes compared to heterosexual and cisgendered communities (Silveri et al. 2022).

The Irish Mental Health Commission produced a guidance paper regarding working with those with LGBTQI+ (Mental Health Commission 2025). The guidance focuses on interpersonal interactions, discussion regarding the avoidance of assumptions and validating gender identities and sexual orientations through use of names, pronouns and identity acknowledgement. The guidance also issues guidance regarding training, education, policies and guidelines, and community engagement (Mental Health Commission 2025). Response to this paper was positive, with Keenan et al. (2026) discussing its importance in providing a roadmap for policy-makers, clinicians and service managers.

Disability, Neurodiversity and Access

Autism Spectrum disorder (ASD) is one of a range of neurodevelopmental conditions defined in the DSM-5 and ICD-11. Autistic people experience significant health disparities and consequently a reduced life expectancy (Doherty et al. 2023). The proportion of the population diagnosed with autism in England has grown significantly over the last few years, and that rate of growth is accelerating further (NHS England 2025a). Authors (Doherty et al. 2023) have created a simple acronym and framework 'SPACE' to support equitable clinical services.

Sensory

Lifelong sensory sensitivities are a diagnostic characteristic of autism (NHS England 2022). There are three categories of autistic sensory sensitivities:

Hyper-sensitivity

- Extreme over-reactivity to sensory input.

Hyposensitivity

- Extreme under-reactivity to sensory input.

Sensory seeking

- Unusual interest in aspects on sensory environment (NHS England 2022).

Sensory interactions can happen across the range of senses, and these are discussed within Table 1 (Doherty et al. 2023).

Table 1 Sensory interactions

Sensation	Considerations	Examples
Sight	Visual sensitivities are common Autistic people can notice visual stimuli such as flickering of lights or computer screens which may go unnoticed by others	Bright lights can be a particular challenge, especially in hospital environments Highly patterned surfaces Overhead rotary fans
Sound	This covers both auditory sensitivities and auditory processing differences. Environmental noises can cause a significant distress to those with a diagnosis of autism, especially those which might be loud or sudden. Autistic people may struggle to hear a conversation in a room that is loud or noisy,	Humming of electrical equipment
Smell	Autistic people may be highly sensitive to sound and may perceive olfactory stimuli. Common and non-offence smells may be perceived as highly troublesome. Some autistic people may be hyposensitive to smell	Coffee
Taste	Autistic people may be hypo- or hyper-sensitive to taste. Autistic people may need highly flavoured or very bland food. Autistic people may like 'same foods' and have a limited and narrow diet.	
Touch	Tactile sensitivities may vary from the inability to tolerate sensations of certain materials to an inability to be touched.	Medical examinations may be more challenging if a person cannot tolerate being touched.
Temperature	Thermal sensitivity is common and lead to out of season clothing.	Tolerated temperatures is likely to be person specific.
Proprioception	This will vary between people.	Some may tend to climb, swing, rock or jump.
Interoception and pain	Some autistic people may have challenges in interpreting internal bodily sensations.	Difficulties in noticing hunger, thirst, tiredness, or a need to urinate or defaecate.

Predictability

Autistic people may need predictability. There may be a preference for routine and structure within those people who have a diagnosis of autism (Doherty et al. 2023). Health environments often offer the complete opposite of predictable environments. Making reasonable adjustments can be useful to make sure you make environments as predictable as possible, and by giving opportunities for service users to visit prior to their appointment.

Acceptance

People with autism need acceptance to be who they are and not have to mask their behaviours. By accepting autistic adults and children, and celebrating their strengths and talents, we can all practise in a way that is more compassionate and understanding (Bristol Autism Support n.d.). There is growing understanding that there are many adults and children with autism, however, there has not necessarily yet been the change in the mainstream for people to accept behaviours in a compassionate and understanding way.

Communication

Autistic people will communicate differently (Doherty et al. 2023). It is important as clinicians that we ensure that we understand and respect that people may communicate differently. People who are autistic may prefer to use more direct language, formal language or echolalia (repeated words and phrases). People who are autistic may find it harder to read facial expressions or body language. They may find it harder to judge pauses or turn-taking in conversations and find it harder to be interrupted whilst in conversation. Always take time to reflect-in-action and consider whether your perceptions of a conversation may be impacted by the differences in how we communicate (National Autistic Society 2025).

Empathy

People with autism may also 'mask'. Masking refers to an autistic person's management of their social presentation to try and minimise or mask their autistic traits from others. Not all autistic people will mask, and those who do mask may not always realise they are doing it. It may be hard for people to stop masking, even if they are consciously trying to not mask. Masking may become a challenge as it may interfere with a person's ability to communicate their distress or symptoms during an appointment with a clinician (NHS England 2023).

Adults diagnosed with autism now represent a significant and fast-growing number of service users supported by mental health services in England (NHS England 2025a).

Language Access and Health Literacy

Reflective Questions

1. What written resources do you give to your patient group?
2. Do you routinely check that people can understand the literature that you are giving?

Health Literacy

In the UK, over seven million adults read or write at a level on or below a 9-year-old, and 43% of adults are unable to understand written health information (NHS England 2025a. The World Health Organization (2025) defines health literacy as:

> Health literacy represents the personal knowledge and competencies that accumulate through daily activities, social interactions and across generations.

There is a strong social gradient in the population, with lower levels of health literacy more common amongst the socially and economically disadvantaged (NHS England 2025a). This means if we do not address health literacy, we actually risk increasing the health inequalities which already exist in the UK (NHS England 2025a). Mental health is linked with poor health literacy (Mantell et al. 2020). However, research suggests that health literacy is understudied in the mental health literature and rarely considered when implementing interventions (Fleary et al. 2022). It is of great importance that we understand that any literature we give out to service users is able to be read and understood by them.

Mental Health Literacy

Mental health literacy refers to the ability to identify different mental health disorders, knowing how to seek mental health support, knowledge of the factors and causes, treatments, professional health available and attitudes that promote help seeking (Jorm et al. 1997). Jorm (2012) argues that by having a good level of mental health literacy, individuals gain skills in how to prevent mental ill health occurring, recognise when a mental health disorder might be developing, access self-help and use mental health first aid skills to help those around them.

There has been work completed in the UK to help improve mental health literacy. The development of 'Mental Health First Aid Courses' offers one way of improving mental health literacy, and initially started in Australia (Henderson 2023). In 2019, the national campaign, Every Mind Matters, was launched to help improve mental health literacy in the general population (Chua et al. 2022). Many health trusts and universities offer access to the 'Mental Health First Aid' courses and these offer a simple and structured way to further improve your mental health skills, especially when supporting colleagues, friends and family.

Key Learning Points

Inclusive health care requires understanding of identity, culture and systematic inequalities. Healthcare practitioners must understand how to recognise and act on racism, stigma and discrimination.

We must tackle the ethnic disparities in mental health services, and that will require us all to act.

There is value in understanding the role culture, spirituality, and religion take in our service user's lives.

Addressing health literacy is important to reducing inequalities. Ensuring we ask questions about people's literacy levels and ability to understand what is being given to them is important to start ensuring inequalities are reduced. We should not be scared to ask these questions.

Conclusion

Inclusive mental health practice is rooted in equity, dignity and an understanding of how social, cultural, and structural factors affect people's lives and experiences of health care. As discussed within this chapter, many groups such as ethnic minorities, LGBTQI+ communities, autistic adults, migrants and people experiencing homelessness face significant barriers to accessing care and often experience poorer outcomes within mental health services. These barriers may include discrimination, stigma, mistrust of services, communication difficulties, financial hardship or previous negative experiences of health care. Healthcare practitioners therefore play a key role in reducing these disparities through culturally responsive practice, accessible communication, trauma-informed approaches and advocacy for systemic change. Building trusting therapeutic relationships and recognising the individuality of each person's experience are essential aspects of inclusive practice.

Inclusive care is much more than knowledge alone. As practitioners, we are required to actively challenge discrimination, prejudice and inequality within the services that we provide. This involves recognising our own assumptions, biases and limitations, whilst remaining open to learning from the experiences of those we support. There have been examples of inequality highlighted throughout this chapter and across this book, demonstrating the real impact that exclusion and inequitable care can have on individuals, families and communities. Practitioners must therefore be willing to reflect critically on their own practice and advocate for environments that promote fairness, accessibility and respect for diversity.

Inclusivity is not an optional aspect of practice but a professional, moral and ethical standard that many of our healthcare registration bodies require of us. It is central to safe, compassionate and person-centred care. All clinicians have the ability and responsibility to contribute to a healthcare system that is safer, more compassionate, and more equitable for every individual who seeks support. Through reflective practice, ongoing education and genuine commitment to equality, healthcare professionals can help create services where all people feel valued, heard and able to access the support they need without fear of judgement or exclusion.

References

Ayaz SS, Asghar-Ali AA (2025) Transcultural Aspects of Mental Health Care. In: Sanches M, Soares JC (eds) Fundamentals of Clinical Psychiatry: A Practical Handbook. Cambridge: Cambridge University Press, pp. 78–85

Bansal N, Karlsen S, Sashidharan SP, Cohen R, Chew-Graham CA, Malpass A (2022) Understanding ethnic inequalities in mental healthcare in the UK: A meta-ethnography. PLoS Med 19(12):e1004139. https://doi.org/10.1371/journal.pmed.1004139. Accessed 24 July 2026

Bignall T, Jeraj S, Helsby E, Butt J (2019) Racial disparities in mental health: literature and evidence review. London: Race Equality Foundation. Available at: https://raceequalityfoundation.org.uk/wp-content/uploads/2022/10/mental-health-report-v5-2.pdf. Accessed 10 May 2026

Bristol Autism Support (n.d.) Autism acceptance. Available at: https://www.bristolautismsupport.org/autism-acceptance/. Accessed 30 Jan 2026

Care Quality Commission (2025) Culturally appropriate care. Available at: https://www.cqc.org.uk/guidance-providers/adult-social-care/culturally-appropriate-care. Accessed 7 May 2026

Chua K-C, Hahn JS, Farrell S, Jolly A, Khangura R, Henderson C (2022) Mental health literacy: a focus on daily life context for population health measurement. SSM Ment Health 2:100118. https://doi.org/10.1016/j.ssmmh.2022.100118. Accessed 14 June 2026

Cochran SD (2001) Emerging issues in research on lesbians' and gay men's mental health: does sexual orientation really matter?. Am Psychol 56(11):931–947. https://doi.org/10.1037/0003-066x.56.11.931. Accessed 18 June 2025

Cook CC (2004) Addiction and spirituality. Addiction 99(5):539–551. https://doi.org/10.1111/j.1360-0443.2004.00715.x. Available from 18 October 2025

Doherty M, McCowan S, Shaw SCK (2023) Autistic SPACE: a novel framework for meeting the needs of autistic people in healthcare settings. Br J Hosp Med 84(4):1–9. Available at: https://doi.org/10.12968/hmed.2023.0006. Accessed 18 June 2025

Equality Act (2010) c. 15. Available at: https://www.legislation.gov.uk/ukpga/2010/15. Accessed 20 July 2026

Fiorillo A, Ventriglio A, Bhugra D (2025) Mental health services around the globe. Int Rev Psychiatry 37:201–202. https://doi.org/10.1080/09540261.2025.2532982. Accessed 18 Nov 2025

Fleary SA, Joseph PL, Gonçalves C, Somogie J, Angeles J (2022) The relationship between health literacy and mental health attitudes and beliefs. Health Lit Res Pract 6(4):e270–e279. https://doi.org/10.3928/24748307-20221018-01. Accessed 21 June 2025

Garssen B, Visser A, Pool G (2021) Does spirituality or religion positively affect mental health? Meta-analysis of longitudinal studies. Int J Psychol Relig 31(1):4–20. https://doi.org/10.1080/10508619.2020.1729570. Accessed 12 Dec 2025

Gearing RE, Lizardi D (2009) Religion and suicide. J Relig Health 48(3):332–341. https://doi.org/10.1007/s10943-008-9181-2. Accessed 12 Jan 2026

Gibson P (1989) Gay male and lesbian youth suicide. In: Feinleib MR (ed) Report of the Secretary's Task Force on youth suicide. Volume 3: Prevention and interventions in youth suicide. U.S. Department of Health and Human Services, Washington, DC, pp 110–142. Available at: https://hamara.org.il/wp-content/uploads/2020/09/גיבסון-פול-התאבדויות-בקרב-צעירים-הומואים-ולסביות-1989.pdf. Accessed 7 May 2026

Henderson C (2023) Challenges in improving mental health literacy at population level. World Psychiatry 22(3):392–393. https://doi.org/10.1002/wps.21115. Accessed 12 Jan 2026

Jorm AF (2012) Mental health literacy: empowering the community to take action for better mental health. Am Psychol 67(3):231–243. https://doi.org/10.1037/a0025957

Jorm AF, Korten AE, Jacomb PA, Christensen H, Rodgers B, Pollitt P (1997) Mental health literacy: a survey of the public's ability to recognise mental disorders and their beliefs about the effectiveness of treatment. Med J Aust 166(4):182–186. https://doi.org/10.5694/j.1326-5377.1997.tb140071.x

Kao LE, Peteet JR, Cook CCH (2020) Spirituality and mental health. J Study Spiritual 10(1):42–54. https://doi.org/10.1080/20440243.2020.1726048

Keenan KM, Barrett E, Higgins A (2026) A critical response to the mental health commission's guidance for staff working in mental health services on the care and treatment of LGBTQIA+ people. Ir J Psychol Med. 43(2):225–227. https://doi.org/10.1017/ipm.2025.10166. Accessed 10 Sept 2025

Larson DB, Sherrill KA, Lyons JS, Craigie FC Jr., Thielman SB, Greenwold MA, Larson SS (1992) Associations between dimensions of religious commitment and mental health reported in the American Journal of Psychiatry and Archives of General Psychiatry: 1978–1989. Am J Psychiatry 149(4):557–559. Available at: https://doi.org/10.1176/ajp.149.4.557. Accessed 19 Feb 2026

Lawrence RE, Oquendo MA, Stanley B (2016) Religion and Suicide Risk: A Systematic Review. Arch Suicide Res 20(1):1–21. https://doi.org/10.1080/13811118.2015.1004494. Accessed 18 Mar 2025

Mantell PK, Annika B, Hildegard C, Stephan R, Christiane W (2020) Peculiarities of health literacy in people with mental disorders: a cross-sectional study. Int J Soc Psychiatry 66:10–22

Mental Health Commission (Ireland) (2025) Guidance for staff working in mental health services on the care and treatment of LGBTQIA+ people. Available at: https://www.mhcirl.ie/sites/default/files/2025-06/MHC%20Guidance%20for%20Staff%20working%20in%20Mental%20Health%20Service%20on%20the%20Care%20and%20Treatment%20of%20LGBTQIA%20%20People.pdf. Accessed 7 May 2026

Mishara BL, Weisstub DN (2016) The legal status of suicide: a global review. Int J Law Psychiatry 44:54–74

Moitra M, Owens S, Hailemariam M, Wilson KS, Mensa-Kwao A, Gonese G, Kamamia CK, White B, Young DM, Collins PY (2023) Global mental health: where we are and where we are going. Curr Psychiatry Rep 25(7):301–311. https://doi.org/10.1007/s11920-023-01426-8. Accessed 15 Mar 2026

Mulongo P, Wainwright J (2024) Championing equalities and addressing vulnerability in mental health care. In: K. M. Wright and M. McKeown, eds. Essentials of Mental Health Nursing. London: SAGE Publications Ltd.

National Autistic Society (2025) Autism and communication. Available at: https://www.autism.org.uk/advice-and-guidance/about-autism/autism-and-communication. Accessed 24 July 2026

National Confidential Inquiry into Suicide and Safety in Mental Health (2026) Annual report: UK and Jersey patient data, 2013–2023. Manchester: The University of Manchester. Available at: NCISH Annual Report 2026. Accessed 18 June 2026

NHS Digital (2021) Mental health statistics annual figures 2020–21. Available at: https://digital.nhs.uk/data-and-information/publications/statistical/mental-health-act-statistics-annual-figures/2020-21-annual-figures Accessed 7 May 2026

NHS England (2022) Meeting the needs of autistic adults in mental health services. Available at: https://www.england.nhs.uk/long-read/meeting-the-needs-of-autistic-adults-in-mental-health-services/. Accessed 7 May 2026

NHS England (2023) A national framework for NHS action on inclusion health. Available at: https://www.england.nhs.uk/long-read/a-national-framework-for-nhs-action-on-inclusion-health/. Accessed 7 May 2026

NHS England (2025a) Health literacy. Available at: https://www.england.nhs.uk/personalisedcare/health-literacy/. Accessed 7 May 2026

NHS England (2025b) Culture of care standards for mental health inpatient services. Available at: https://www.england.nhs.uk/long-read/culture-of-care-standards-for-mental-health-inpatient-services/. Accessed 7 May 2026

Nursing and Midwifery Council (2021) Equity, diversity and inclusion. Available at: https://www.nmc.org.uk/about-us/equity-diversity-and-inclusion/. Accessed 8 June 2025

Rethink Mental Illness (2025) Ethnic minorities and mental health. Available at: https://www.rethink.org/advice-and-information/living-with-mental-illness/ethnic-minorities-immigration-and-mental-health/ethnic-minorities-and-mental-health/. Accessed 7 May 2026

Rosmarin DH, Koenig HG (2020) Handbook of spirituality, religion, and mental health. Academic Press, Cambridge, MA

Silveri G, Schimmenti S, Prina E, Gios L, Mirandola M, Converti M, Fiorillo A, Pinna F, Ventriglio A, Galeazzi GM, Sherriff N, Zeeman L, Amaddeo F, Italian Working Group on LGBTQI Mental Health (2022) Barriers in care pathways and unmet mental health needs in LGBTIQ + communities. International review of psychiatry (Abingdon, England), 34(3–4), 215–229. https://doi.org/10.1080/09540261.2022.2075256. Accessed 21 Mar 2026

Substance Abuse and Mental Health Services Administration (2015) Trauma-informed care in behavioral health services: Quick guide for clinicians (based on TIP 57) (SMA 15–4912). Rockville, MD: Substance Abuse and Mental Health Services Administration. Available at: https://library.samhsa.gov/sites/default/files/sma15-4912.pdf. Accessed 16 Mar 2025

The Guardian (2004) Death of black patient showed up race bias. The Guardian, 6 February. Available at: https://www.theguardian.com/uk/2004/feb/06/race.politics. Accessed 7 May 2026

Tomlinson J, Glenn ES, Paine DR, Sandage SJ (2016) What is the "relational" in relational spirituality? A review of definitions and research directions. J Spiritual Ment Health 18(1):55–75

UN Human Rights Office of the High Commissioner (1992) Declaration on the rights of persons belonging to national or ethnic, religious and linguistic minorities. Available at: https://www.ohchr.org. Accessed 7 May 2026

Weziak-Bialowolska D, Lee MT, Bialowolski P, Chen Y, Vander Weele TJ, McNeely E (2023) Prospective associations between strengths of moral character and health: longitudinal evidence from survey and insurance claims data. Soc Psychiatry Psychiatr Epidemiol 58(1):163–176. https://doi.org/10.1007/s00127-022-02344-5. Accessed 12 Dec 2025

World Health Organization (2021) Improving LGBTIQ+ health and well-being with consideration for SOGIESC. Available at: https://www.who.int/activities/improving-lgbtqi-health-and-well–being-with-consideration-for-sogiesc. Accessed 19 July 2026

World Health Organization (2025) Health literacy. Available at: https://www.who.int/news-room/fact-sheets/detail/health-literacy. Accessed 8 June 2026

Wylie L, Van Meyel R, Harder H, Sukhera J, Luc C, Ganjavi H, Elfakhani M, Wardrop N (2018) Assessing trauma in a transcultural context: challenges in mental health care with immigrants and refugees. Public Health Rev 39:22. https://doi.org/10.1186/s40985-018-0102-y. Accessed 24 July 2026

GPSR Compliance

The European Union's (EU) General Product Safety Regulation (GPSR) is a set of rules that requires consumer products to be safe and our obligations to ensure this.

If you have any concerns about our products, you can contact us on ProductSafety@springernature.com

In case Publisher is established outside the EU, the EU authorized representative is:

Springer Nature Customer Service Center GmbH
Europaplatz 3
69115 Heidelberg, Germany

Batch number: 10791480

Printed by Printforce, the Netherlands